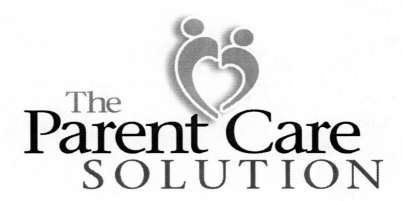

The
Parent Care
SOLUTION

A Legacy of Love...

DAN TAYLOR

authorHOUSE

1663 LIBERTY DRIVE, SUITE 200
BLOOMINGTON, INDIANA 47403
(800) 839-8640
www.authorhouse.com

First published by AuthorHouse 06/07/04

ISBN: 1-4184-7111-9 (sc)
ISBN: 1-4184-6973-4 (dj)

Library of Congress Number: 2004093837

Printed in the United States of America
Bloomington, Indiana

This book is printed on acid-free paper.

SPECIAL TRADEMARK NOTIFICATION
*The Strategic Coach has allowed through written agreement and a special license agreement to integrate certain Strategic Coach concepts into The Parent Care Solution™.

The R-Factor Question™, The D.O.S. Conversation™, Always Increase Your Confidence™ are all trademark terms and the intellectual property of The Strategic Coach, Inc. and are only used in integration with The Parent Care Solution and by specific written permission under license from The Strategic Coach, Inc.

All questions concerning the authorized use of The Strategic Coach concepts should be directed to:

The Strategic Coach, Inc.
33 Fraser Avenue
Toronto, Ontario, Canada
416-531-7399 or 800-387-3206
www.strategiccoach.com

CONTENTS

*This book is dedicated
to my father, Clyde J. Taylor,
and families everywhere.*

CHAPTER ONE

No One Left Behind

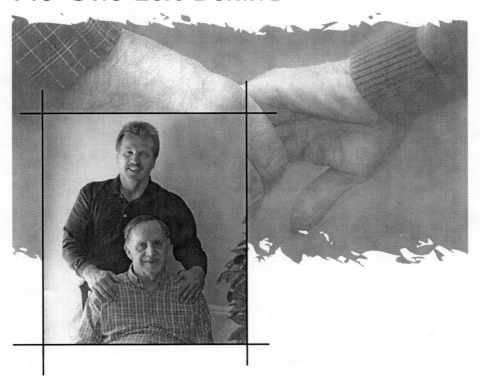

On a pre-spring Sunday in April of 2000 I received a strange phone call concerning my father. On the other end of the phone was a friend of our family who relayed to me that my father was in the protective custody of the police in Danville, Virginia, a small town approximately 100 miles north of Winston-Salem, North Carolina, my father's home. The police had pulled him over for driving erratically at 4:30 in the morning. It seemed that he was disoriented and confused and from all reports had been driving for some time.

When I finally arrived he seemed a bit nonchalant about the

entire matter…sort of as if he had forgotten to shut the kitchen door or perhaps left the light on in the car. Little did I know that he was nonchalant because in his mind nothing had happened worth remembering…in fact he didn't remember anything about the incident. The only thing that he thought strange was that it was Tuesday now and his son almost never came to see him on Tuesday.

On Thursday of that week we left his friend's home and drove together to an appointment with a gerontologist at the Stix Center, Baptist Hospital Winston-Salem, NC. The Stix Center has developed a national reputation for their work in gerontology, aging and seniors care. I was grateful that day for their Critical Assessment and I remain grateful to this day. Although if I had known what the next few years were going to bring, I may have been less than starry-eyed at their ability.

I was grateful that day for their Critical Assessment and I remain grateful to this day.

During the nearly 4 hour assessment my father was given a battery of mental, neuropsychological, physical, and emotional evaluations designed to pinpoint the cause of his rather bizarre behavior.

After what seemed an endless afternoon in the waiting room, the young doctor came out and asked if he could speak with me. He introduced himself with all the calmness that physicians, clergy, and prison wardens exhibit when the news they have to speak is not the news you want to hear, nor could ever imagine.

It seems my father was suffering from late stage dementia (he had been progressively forgetful for almost 5 years) and was in fact in the early stages of Alzheimer's disease. He explained what had happened with the driving incident. Dad had simply turned left instead of right or perhaps forgot where he was going and simply drove as if that is what he had intended to do in the first place.

He continued for the next 15 minutes or so explaining all the signs and symptoms of Alzheimer's, the progression of the disease, and the realistic outcome the family could expect. In retrospect I listened with the sort of numbness that a ballplayer might feel listening to his coach send him back to the huddle with a play when two minutes before he had been clotheslined by someone twice his size.

In his closing remarks he said; "Your father is fine but he cannot live alone or drive his car again." In my numbed naivety I asked, "From what point?" The young doctor with all the patience of one who deals with the mentally ill on a daily basis replied, "Why, from right now."

That afternoon on the Thursday before Palm Sunday in the year of our Lord 2000, the intergenerational transfer of power, wealth, and influence of the Taylor family of Winston-Salem, NC happened in an instant. My father became my child and I became his parent.

The next 5 days were a blur of action, reaction, shock, anger, denial, disbelief, depression, rage, elation, sadness, pain and fatigue.

Looking back, I'm not sure how we made it through those 5 days without permanently damaging everything we held dear.

I phoned my companion of 9 years, Christine, to tell her that I was bringing him home for a few days until we could sort things out and that she should let Ashley, her 14 year old, know that I was coming, as well as our two dogs, two cats, and whoever or whatever happened to be in our home at the time.

Our home in Charlotte, NC is a 4,200 square foot three story stucco with swimming pool, lots of stairs, original art and nothing at all to make a 74-year-old retired railroad foreman feel comfortable. I had no idea that the décor incompatibility would be the least of our concerns.

When we arrived, I helped my father downstairs to our library/theatre, dog-sleeping place, and walkout to the pool basement of our house. Most of that Thursday was spent making small talk, fixing assorted meals, and when he didn't see me, sneaking into Chris' office to cry about the entire situation. I lost count of the visits to that office over the weekend.

That night I had to bathe, dress, shave, and generally get him ready for bed. Any modesty for either of us was quickly dispensed with as we both intuitively knew what I had to do. He had to let me do what he could no longer do or remember to do for himself. I slept with the proverbial one eye open as I listened for him to get up, miss the bathroom and trip down the stairs to be impaled on some blown glass flower in the hallway.

When morning finally came, I began what was to be the ritual for the next 5 days of newspaper small talk, coffee, two

eggs and bacon, an assisted bowel movement and the beginning
of a day of news, talk shows, and repetitive stares.

Sometime about 1pm on Good Friday, it occurred to me that
I had to be in Florida the next Wednesday on business and that
I truly, really, really truly, honest to goodness had no plan B for
his care – It further occurred to me that unless I found a
solution to this dilemma I would have more than parent care
issues to deal with when I returned.

With all the confidence that comes with ignorance, I began
phoning nursing homes, geriatric centers, retirement homes (I
thought they were all the same) to inquire whether there might
be room at some inn for my father. Since I had never been faced
with this before, I assumed you just drove up, weekend bag in
hand with proof of insurability, a pure heart, and a small down
payment and Dad would be greeted, treated, and checked right
on in much like a Four Seasons visit.

The next six hours were like a visit to Dante's Circles of
Special Care hell. Not only did I not know the questions to ask,
I didn't know the language, culture, or cause dé existence for
assisted living centers. I likened it to a first visit to France where
what I wanted to visit was the Eiffel Tower, the French refused
to speak English and the only words I knew were "please" and
"croissant".

A lawyer by training, financial advisor by occupation, and
genetically an entrepreneur, I have always prided myself on my
ability to out-think, out-innovate, and out-perform any set of
obstacles, challenges, or difficulties placed in my path. By the

end of the afternoon I had gotten some of the language, understood a little of what I needed to know and do, and made an appointment with a center in Charlotte and one in Winston-Salem. They represented that if we worked diligently we could have my dad safe and sound in his new facility by Monday evening.

While those visits are the stories for another chapter, let me just say that what was to follow after the facility decision made the facility decision seem like someone had asked if I wanted fries with my order.

After a restless Easter Sunday filled with a hurriedly assembled Easter basket, faux joviality and the myopic conversation that occurs between father and son when there is no more small talk or superficial subjects to discuss; Monday and transport time arrived.

Whether my Father knew he was going to a new place to live or not, I don't know and will probably never know. What I do know and acutely remember is that I knew and was completely aware that my life and my father's would never be the same.

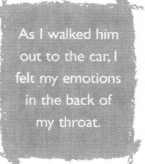

As I walked him out to the car, I felt my emotions in the back of my throat.

As I walked him out to the car, I felt my emotions in the back of my throat. I helped him in, fastened his seat belt and mumbled some excuse about having to go back in to get something.

As I opened the door and shut it quickly, Christine came into the foyer and asked, "What's wrong?" The pent-up emotions of the past 5 days came out in a torrent of tears and gut wrenching sobs. I cried out that I could not do this and fell on my knees in a flood of tears, rage, and frustration over what had happened.

I cried for a few minutes longer, took another few moments to get myself together and walked back out to my car to begin the two-hour ride to the Village Care facility in King, NC.

During the next two hours my father told me the same story six times and I listened on the sixth time with the same level of attention that I did the first time. It was my sixth time hearing it but each time it was his first time telling it. I remember thinking that this must be what living in a mental institution is like.

We arrived and began the in processing that is specific to every facility like this in the United States. My father was not sure why he was there; all he knew was that all he wanted was to go home and to have me take him.

I lied that day to my father. The only lie I have ever told him. I lied that he was there for a check-up and that we would go home a little bit later. By the time later came, he had forgotten not only the lie, but where he was and where home might be.

As I settled him into his room, I realized I had forgotten a couple of things from his home nearby that might make him more comfortable. Things like pictures, his favorite shirt, and his table radio. I explained to him where I was going and asked him if there was anything else special he would like while the doctors were checking him out.

He said, "I want my two caps." Surprised at the specificity of the response, I asked him which two caps out of his cap collection that he wanted. He said that he wanted his Shriner's cap, my father is a life-long Mason in a family of Masons and I knew that cap would give him some security. "What's the other cap, Dad?" I asked. He said, "I want the Navy SEAL cap." My dad, who had been in the Navy, but never a SEAL had somehow gotten a cap with the SEAL lettering. Curious, I asked, "Why do you want the Navy SEAL cap?" He replied, "Because the SEALs never leave anyone behind…and I know you won't leave me behind."

This is a book about not leaving someone behind. More importantly, it's a book about how to have the conversations, make the plans, and extend the relationship with the most important people you have ever been in relationship with, your parents. It is a book about how to think, communicate, and take action for the inevitable time when your parents are no longer able or willing to be responsible for themselves. It is a book about how to begin a conversation that deepens over time about deep things with two people who brought you to the planet. At the risk of being cheesy, it ends in love what began in love and that is the caring, nurturing, and protection of parent with child and child with a parent.

It is a book primarily about the conversations you need to have and secondarily about the solutions you need to implement. Whether the solution is a care facility, a caregiver, or a long-term care policy, life insurance contract or power of attorney, the "How" becomes much more obvious after we discover the "What".

The "How" can be arranged through the almost infinite number of lawyers, accountants, financial planners, investment advisors and the like whose business and expertise is the recommendation of specific solutions.

The "What" is a little bit more complicated. What are the things you need to talk about? What are the things you need to decide? What are the things you need to do? What are the changes you need to make? What are the things to be scared about? What are the things to be excited about? What are the advantages that you have? What are the things you want to say and what are the things you want to be said…between you, about you, for you, with them - your parents.

The Parent Care Solution™ is a Unique Process* that focuses on the Six Critical Conversations to have with your parents or about your parents if you anticipate a role in decisions about their future care. If you are parents, it is a process that you enter into with your spouse or third party about your future care whether your children are involved or not. It is a conversation architecture designed to build something that reflects contemplation, restores relationship, and creates confidence for all who use it.

> It is a conversation architecture designed to build something that reflects contemplation, restores relationship, and creates confidence for all who use it.

The Parent Care Solution™ is a model that is totally adaptable, totally flexible, and totally capable of evolving and changing with your situation. I have no preconceived idea about how it expands, where it goes, how it evolves or deepens. I only have a desire that it be used, a hope that it will and a belief that had someone had this process in place for 5 days in the early spring of 2000 that I would have spent less time on the phone and with forms and more time in conversation and care with the one who needed these things. My hope is that you will find it helpful on your journey.

CHAPTER TWO

The Relationship Time Bomb

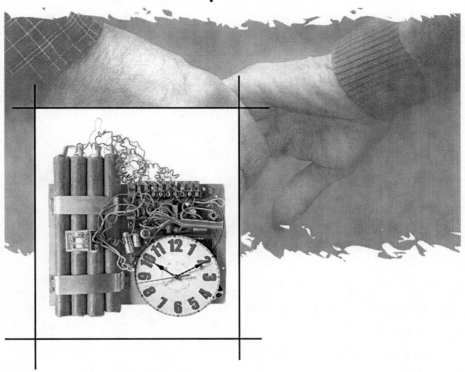

On January 1, 1996 the first Baby-Boomer turned age 50. By January 1, 2010 the Boomers will begin transforming to the largest population of the elderly in the history of the world. It is estimated that between 2011 and 2030 the numbers of elderly will grow from 40 million to 70+ million and will continue to climb.

Ken Dychwald in his groundbreaking works on aging; *Age Wave* and *Age Power* brilliantly structures the major issues those statistics will force us to live, work and reconsider.

1. More of us will live longer than any previous generation.

In all likelihood we will spend more time taking care of our parents than we did in raising our children.

2. The epicenter of economic and political power will shift from young to old. The AARP is the second largest non-profit in the world, ranking only behind the Catholic Church, and having more members than the NAACP, NRA, Boy Scouts, National PTA, AFL-CIO, and League of Women Voters combined.

3. We will need to change our current mind-set about how to spend our extra years in life. NONE of the existing financial, medical, vocational or community structures support the outdated notions of detachment, decline, or disengagement that retirement at age 65 creates.

4. How we decide to behave as elders will in all likelihood be the most important challenge we face in our lives. We are about to enter the perfect storm of inter-generational relationships: The Best Generation, The Boomer Generation, and Generation X all thrown together in a melting pot of conflicting goals, resources, and priorities. While the intermingling of these generations takes the form of a triangle, the coming together will really create more of a relationship time bomb.

> How we decide to behave as elders will in all likelihood be the most important challenge we face in our lives.

While it's tempting at this point to launch into a few dozen pages of statistics, graphs, and charts to illustrate the evidence that the wealthiest, most well-educated, most experienced group of people ever assembled on the planet will soon be turning into caretakers for their parents, it really isn't necessary. Just as the post-World War II society was not prepared for the huge numbers in the Baby Boom Generation, the Baby Boom Generation is not prepared for all the things that will be required of it as it attempts to take care of its parents while at the same time creating its own care.

The Baby Boom Generation changed the existing relationships of a number of societal structures when it began to exercise its demographic muscle. School systems, neighborhoods, employers, health care, and government were all deluged at the same time with what can be summarized as a common request for more: more schools, teachers, and higher education opportunities. More housing, cars, and accessories. More jobs, business opportunities, and the money required for both of them. More say in the how local, state, and federal government structured the rules of daily lives.

What happened from 1945-1960 is on the verge of happening again with different kinds of demands of more. This time the more is centered around life extending/enhancing solutions, instead of life creation/design proposals. The "more" that the Boomer Generation requires this time has to do with getting older, not being younger.

The "more" takes many forms: more and better-personalized, and responsive health care. More and better-personalized, flexible and adaptive housing.

More and better-personalized, unique and relevant employment opportunities. More and better-personalized, creative and evolutionary financial tools and strategies for a generation that will ultimately be more concerned about the inadequacy of its own retirement than the loss of its inheritance.

Not withstanding all of those requests for more, this is not a book about the "How To's" of solving those "more" problems. This is a book about how to create a conversation with or on behalf of your parents or with or on behalf of your children. It is a book about creating a relationship through a series of conversations that allow you to talk about the specific, tactical, solutions to the "more" issues inside a larger context.

The great challenge facing the Baby Boom Generation and their parents as well as the mutual challenges and opportunities for their aging parents is that neither the Boomers nor their parents know how to begin the conversations that could identify the dangers, the opportunities, and the advantages that each generation has. The conversations are important for both sides because without the relationship that the conversations create, all you have is a series of partitioned and disconnected transaction communications that force-feed the need for some type of quick-fix solution.

...the conversation offered in *The Parent Care Solution* is one that creates relationship by establishing communication, collaboration, and clarity...

Instead, the conversation offered in *The Parent Care Solution* is one that creates relationship by establishing communication, collaboration, and clarity around all these aging issues. The relationship is critical in helping to resolve the mutual problems facing parents and children because the conversation about care is just one of the relationship conversations that you may be required to have with, or on behalf of your parents.

While *The Parent Care Solution* has limited itself to relationship conversations around the basics for preparation for long-term care there are any number of relationship conversations that demand an opportunity to be heard. There is the relationship that you and your parents have around lifestyle. The relationship around profession or opportunity. There's the one around health and medical needs. Finally, there is the relationship around death and dying.

The friction that may occur between the Best Generation, the Boomer Generation, and the X Generation as they try to resolve their mutual challenges of interdependency with everything from the environment, health care and the job market is really more of an opportunity for alignment than a cause for alienation. The obvious statement about all of this can really be boiled down to 3 thoughts:

- **We are all here together**
- **Nobody gets through unless we all do**
- **We can do this by default or design**

The Parent Care Solution favors design over default. Inherent in its structure is the belief that what people want more than anything, especially in this age and time is an opportunity for community, conversation, and collaboration.

Will *The Parent Care Solution* work for all of the Baby Boomers and their parents, a sort of psychological Swiss Army knife for the relationship campground? Probably not. Why you ask? There are as many reasons why it won't work, as there are people who won't use it. But that really isn't and shouldn't be your focus. Why someone else won't use *The Parent Care Solution* or why it didn't work for them is not relevant to you and your situation at all.

What is relevant is whether it works for you. Here's how you find out if it will. Try it.

CHAPTER THREE

The Big Picture Question

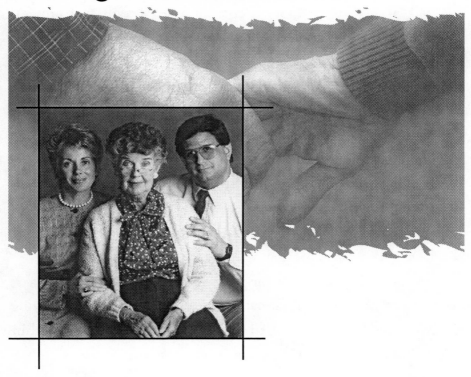

It may seem counter-intuitive that the key to *The Parent Care Solution* is not a product in the ordinary sense at all. Rather, the products one would ordinarily expect in a conversation about parent care: nursing homes, annuities, assisted living centers, life insurance, caregivers, etc. are, in my model, implementation tools designed to *support* a structure of care rather than *create* a structure of care. Let me explain.

The typical financial services, insurance industry, or CPA firm approach to parent care begins with the introduction of a product that purports to be part or all of the solution to this parent care problem. If you've chatted with a lawyer the solution is a will, perhaps a trust, or other sorts of legal tools that protect assets, enrich beneficiaries, and allow an extension of your legal rights and powers through a third party or a personal representative, General Power of Attorney or Healthcare Power of Attorney. The patient care problem is a legal one and these are the tools used to solve legal problems.

The investment profession's approach to the parent care solution is an accumulation model favoring growth and income over pure growth, cross-correlated with various markets, exchanges and indexes, weighted against one's risk profile and sensitivity to volatility. The emphasis is on some form of preservation of capital that purports to preserve purchasing power, partly allow for reasonable withdrawals, while still leaving a tidy sum to beneficiaries. All of this of course occurring within a complex conundrum of economic, tax, interest rate, and global commerce environments, which in some form or another affects the model. One needs only to sit through one of these presentations with a client to understand how afterwards you just decide to spend it all and go straight to the cat food as an appetizer.

The insurance industry approach is only minimally less confusing and somewhat less powerful – the parent care solution here begins with a conversation about long-term care costs, available assets, social security contributions, pension benefits and the minimization of any estate tax with artfully structured individual or second-to-die life insurance. The answer here, like the investment industry is really to just choose some financial tool, let it work its magic, or review it on an annual basis or when events dictate and be ready to reap the windfall.

The accounting industry tends to focus on the various state and federal regulations that affect the purchase and use of products from the investment and insurance industries and the tax ramifications of those decisions. There are titillating conversations over the use of qualified vs. non-qualified monies, social security taxation potential, IRA withdrawal tax traps and whether or not there will be a sunrise after the sunset of current estate tax legislation.

An individual visit to one of the industry practitioners may leave one somewhat confused about the options and with an increased lack of self-confidence about considering the many possibilities. It's overwhelming and enough to make you decide to think

> An individual visit to one of the industry practitioners may leave one somewhat confused...

about it another day (which by the way never comes) when your head isn't hurting so badly and the suicidal impulses subside.

Here's the problem with all of these industries and their response to the parent care dilemma: It isn't that the industries are bad. It isn't that they are not populated with bright, well-intentioned, learned practitioners. It isn't that the solutions that they offer are inappropriate. In fact, it isn't about the products those industries offer at all. The fact is, you have to use some sampling of those products otherwise no kind of solution can be implemented no matter which profession offers it.

The problem is simply this. All the industries and professions are providing a *product solution* to what is first and foremost a *process problem*. The process problem is not about the solution to the problem, it's about the conversation about the problem. The problem in parent care is the conversation about parent care: *with* Baby Boomers and their parents, with Baby Boomers *about* their parents, *with parents* about their Baby Boomers and *with everybody* in a room talking with each other about this.

The reality of all this is that once you know the "What" of what needs to be done, the "How" to do it becomes relatively easy. The focus of this book is the "What" conversation. The "How" of that conversation then becomes a matter of available resources and available capabilities, when you have them, when you need them.

Don't misunderstand me here. I have spent the last 20+ years around lawyers, accountants, financial planners, stockbrokers, and insurance sales people. For most of those 20 years I have practiced with them, collaborated with them, and competed against them as we built our advisory business. It's not that those industries and those products are inappropriate. They are appropriate in and of themselves. The problem is that they are introduced in an inappropriate and premature manner for the Baby Boom Generation and their parents.

What the Baby Boomers and their parents are looking for in the parent care problem is not a product, but a process. And the process is not about the conversation about which product to choose. It is a conversation about what kind of support to provide for their parents, how they create that support, and how they solve some of the challenges that the support requires.

Shoshanna Zuboff in her book, *The Support Economy* says that what the Baby Boom Generation is looking for is not another product presentation but a conversation around what she says is their desire to establish a system of deep support that allows them to accomplish their goals of psychological self-determination.

> The creative marketing psychology of managerial capitalism was to create a desire, identification, and dependence...

Zuboff says that the old world of managerial capitalism, that is industries that were designed around the manufacture, distribution and service of mass-produced products, is still necessary but woefully inadequate to meet the psychological and deep support needs of the most intelligent, affluent, self-aware, and well educated generation of people in the industry of the world. The creative marketing psychology of managerial capitalism was to create a desire, identification, and dependence on the products (non-commodities) that managers of those capitalistic systems produced.

Her point is this – what the consumer does not want is more choices. Whether it's the 63 models of SUV available, the 9,000 separate mutual funds or the 15 different kinds of deep-dish pizza. There are already too many choices and options.

She says that what the 21st century consumer wants is in actuality a set of relationships that produce a system of deep support that allows the consumer to ascend to higher levels of what she labels, psychological self-determination: I want what I want when I want it, in the way that I want it and whoever provides it has to assume total accountability and responsibility for the consumption experience surrounding it. Deep support is about allowing the 21st century consumer to maximize the experience in relation to their goals and desires as opposed to being affected by the products of consumption in unpredictable ways with unintended consequences.

It is *The Parent Care Solution* that provides the beginning of this experience of deep support for both the Baby Boomers and their parents. It is *The Parent Care Solution* that creates the psychological self-determination structure that makes the legal, accounting, brokerage, insurance, and care industries' products more of a fait accompli decision instead of a driving force decision. In other words, once you determine the type of deep support that is desired and the type of deep support that can be provided, the selection of the various professional, financial, or investment products is, sad to say, relatively an easy matrix of decisions.

The Parent Care Solution begins with something we call **The Parent Care Conversations**. The Parent Care Conversations are *six* specifically designed conversations that focus on the primary areas of deep support that must be addressed to accomplish a high level of psychological self-determination. The Parent Care Conversations are: The Big Picture Conversation, The House Conversation, The Money Conversation, The Care Conversation, The Property Conversation, and The Legacy Conversation. The Parent Care Conversations are cumulative in nature and inherently conflict resolving. They are designed to discover in each area what our parents are most concerned about, what they are most excited about, and what strengths or advantages they bring to each situation to help them minimize their concerns, maximize their opportunities, and reinforce their strengths. There are no preconceived ideas in these conversations about any problems or any solutions. Nor are there preconceived ideas about excitements or advantages. There are only the questions and the answers to them.

The Parent Care Conversations are prefaced by an introductory conversation that we call **The Parent Care Big Picture Question**. The Parent Care Big Picture Question is a variation of a tool I have used in my advisory practice for years and was designed by Dan Sullivan, the creator and founder of The Strategic Coach Program. The tool is called The R-Factor Question* and is part of the The D.O.S. Conversation*. It is used here with permission from The Strategic Coach Inc.

More information on The D.O.S. Conversation* as well as other Strategic Coach programs and products can be found at www.strategiccoach.com.

The Parent Care Big Picture Question is simply this: **"If we were sitting here in this same time and place**

3 years from now and looking back, what has to have happened for you to feel good about all your decisions concerning your long term care?"

The reason this question is so important to ask is that it gives you insight about your parents' (1) ideas about how they view their future care and (2) whether they trust you enough to discuss it with you. If your parents have not, will not, or cannot bring themselves to think about their long-term care from a conceptual standpoint, you have a huge challenge ahead of you. If they cannot or will not trust you enough to discuss the view they have, then you have an impossible task. You cannot participate or be held responsible for your parents' care unless you can be part of a conversation about their care. It is really that simple.

> You cannot participate or be held responsible for your parents' care unless you can be part of a conversation about their care.

The next three questions in The Parent Care Big Picture Questions are based on the remaining questions from The D.O.S. Conversation* modified for your parents. In The D.O.S. Conversation* you are attempting to discover what your parents' dangers, opportunities, and strengths are concerning their long-term care. The D.O.S. Conversation for your parents in this situation would look like this:

"If we were to look forward to 3 years from now, what are some of the fears that you have with these long-term care decisions?" (Dangers)

"If we were to look forward 3 years from now, what are some of the things that excite you about these long-term care decisions?" (Opportunities)

"What are the strengths or advantages that you think you bring to these decisions to help you minimize the things you are afraid of and maximize the things you are excited about?" (Strengths)

The answers to these questions provide the basis for your early conversations and the context in which all of the conversations take place. As you read through the rest of the conversations you will see how each question and the ensuing answers help you to create the picture of care that your parents would like you to see.

CHAPTER FOUR

The Money Conversation

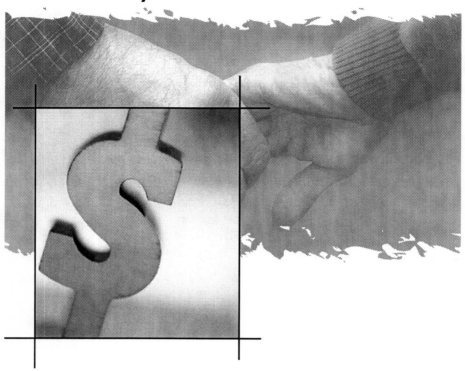

The Money Conversation is our name for the process that you use to do an inventory of all the financial assets that your parents have so that you can determine any number of things important for planning the future:

1. **How much they have**
2. **How much they owe**
3. **What is working**
4. **What isn't working**
5. **What we want to change**

If your parents are the rule and not the exception they

probably have a little bit of everything financial tucked in a variety of places with any number of advisors. **The goal with The Money Conversation is to (1) get an understanding of what your parents understand about what they have and (2) to get specific financial information to verify those understandings.**

The information gathering forms can be used to create clarity or madness depending on how you use them. If you choose to complete them by yourself, try not to begin and end the information gathering piece making your parents feel like they've just been invited to participate in an interrogation scene out of "Law and Order". If you work with a Parent Care Specialist™, he, or she, has been specifically trained to gather the information in a way that is open and inviting and not threatening, judgmental or embarrassing.

In the United States the amount of money we have at the end of our career is judged by some to be a measure of the success of our life's work. If your parents grew up in the depression or pre-World War II they have the emotional hangover from the worst financial disaster in history. For many people of that generation there will never be enough of anything to make them feel secure financially. They are fearful of growing old without money, without a place to live, and unable to afford to eat or visit their grandkids. Part of the reluctance to discuss money with this generation is a reluctance to discuss the possibility of financial failure. Money is a private thing, talked about in private, counted in private and given away in private.

Your parents may feel that they have not done well enough and are embarrassed to share that with you. They may feel that they have done so well that if they gave you a peek at what you might inherit you would quit your job, throw caution to the wind, build up inventories of tanning oil and sunglasses, and generally join the ranks of the world's nare-do-wells.

No matter how you view it, or talk about it, money is not the easiest topic to have a conversation about. The D.O.S. Conversation* makes the transition a bit easier in that you are asking them to describe what the future looks like if they have made decisions about their long-term care. Their answer is almost a fait accompli to discussing certain financial issues. When you discuss the things they are afraid of, the things they are excited about, and the strengths they bring to the situation, it somehow makes the gathering of the financial information a set of mental exercises instead of the equivalent of a tax audit.

You might consider gathering this information in two phases. The first phase is what I call The Money Information™. You're attempting to find out as much as you can instead of every little detail about every little thing. After you've gathered the personal information, ask them if they would mind to give you the latest copies of information they have about everything.

After you get the statements, you can record things like asset location, account numbers, amounts, ownership, and other information. Your job is to put together a complete picture of where they are; understand it may take just a little time to do this. Your parents didn't accumulate all they have in one night and you aren't going to understand it in one night.

If you choose to work with a Parent Care Specialist, he or she will have been specifically trained to gather this information in a way that facilitates the communication between you and your parents and deepens the connection, hence the trust. Trust is not necessarily based on the time that people spend together. People can spend a lifetime together and never trust each other. Trust is more about intensity and focus of interest. This conversation about money can be very intense, very intimate, and very revealing. It has been our experience that if you can have this conversation, you can have the other conversations much easier.

> People can spend a lifetime together and never trust each other.

You have to have this conversation because you have to know what you're working with from a financial point of view. You cannot begin to select a care facility until you understand what you are able to pay on a monthly basis for that facility. You won't understand whether the family home is an asset or a liability until you have this conversation. You will not understand whether you can disregard the social security income or whether you must totally depend on it. You can't give the Old Masters away until you understand that you won't need to trade them for the cash to live on.

Whatever the picture that's created, whatever you find out, it will be helpful in designing the solution. You cannot create more than there is there in most cases, but you must, in most cases, use all that is there.

When you've gathered all the information, there are probably 50 different ways and 10,000 different opinions on how to use it. The numbers of scenarios that you can imagine are simply mind-boggling. How is one to decide how to do what first?

At the risk of seeming overly simplistic, we have designed something that we call Easy Money, Hard Money™. Here's how it works:

Easy Money is that money that:
1. Is easily gotten
2. Is easily transferred
3. Has little or no tax effect
4. Does not effect long-term growth

Hard Money is money that:
1. Is difficult to convert to Easy Money
2. Is not quickly or easily sold
3. Has a tax bill attached to its sale
4. Ends the potential for long-term gain

At the risk of going against prevailing wisdom, our bet is to go with Easy Money first and Hard Money last, all things being equal.

Be careful here to not get lost in all the financial modeling tools available. There are financial software tools that will help you create a model portfolio based on a multitude of scenarios and factors. While interesting from an intellectual standpoint and fun from a "Money as Play Station™" in the end one is still left (1) understanding what is going on today and (2) trying to guess what will happen tomorrow.

Here's how to do this without going completely bonkers. Develop a worst-case, real case, best-case viewpoint to plan for care:

Worst Case – What the 100 year history of earnings has been in the markets minus 50% (about 4% to 5%).

Real Case – What the 100 year history of earnings has equaled (around 9% to 10%).

Best Case – What the 100 year history of earnings has been plus 3% to 5% (about 12% to 15%).

Assume also that you will preserve as much principle as possible. In other words, your parents will not die broke. Assume also that the cost of your parents' care will increase the same way: worst case, real case, best case.

What you're trying to arrive at here is a number that you can more or less use to get a feeling for how long your parents can stay in a facility without (a) beginning to eat into principle or (b) going completely broke.

Your Parent Care Specialist has been trained to gather this information, analyze this information, and give you the best recommendation based on years of experience and wisdom. Don't take their observations and recommendations as the absolute truth. They're making educated guesses the same way that you would except at a higher and hopefully more integrated level.

THE MONEY CONVERSATION

R-Factor Question*	If we were sitting here in this same time and place a year from now and looking back, what decisions about your money in relation to your long-term care do you have to have made to feel **good** about your progress?
D.	If we were to look forward over the next year at the money decision, what is it that you find **fearful** about making this decision?
O.	If we were to look forward over the next year at the money decisions, what is it that you find **exciting** about making this decision?
S.	What is it, in the form of strengths or advantages that you bring to these decisions to help **minimize** the things that scare you and **maximize** the things that excite you?

THE MONEY CONVERSATION
Answers

D. **DANGERS**

- Don't have enough, don't know it
- Don't know where everything is
- Don't know how to organize it
- Don't know what I'm earning
- Don't know how it should be organized
- Will run out of money too soon
- Will live too long for money
- Don't know where I should be investing
- Don't know how to decide

O. **OPPORTUNITIES**

- Can get financial affairs organized
- Can maximize earnings potential
- Can take profits where needed
- Can diversify for protection
- Can delegate to professionals
- Can make sure money lasts
- Can maximize money to children
- Can assure finances for long-term care

S. **STRENGTHS**

- Have or can get financial resources
- Have prepared financially, emotionally for decision
- Have evaluated best possible care options
- Family is in support of idea
- Am ready for transition
- Some of my friends have already made this decision
- Have always been easily adaptable in new situations
- I understand all the consequences of my decision

CHAPTER FIVE

The House Conversation

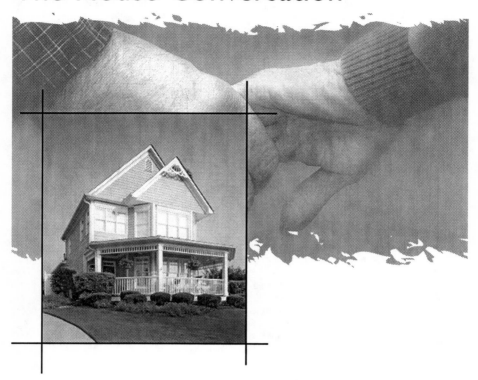

I think **The House Conversation** is perhaps the most potentially emotional and conflicted conversation that you will have with your parents. The axiom, a man's home is his castle, is also in the 21st century, true for women as well.

Whether the home you're talking to them about is part of a family estate that has been passed down for years or the patio golf course dwelling, it still represents at a symbolic level independence, autonomy, control, status, and a final fortress to play "me against the world".

For people who have been in the same house for years, the

family home is full of memories. It's the place where new babies came to, where Santa visited, where grandma spent some time. It is the site of lots of firsts in people's lives. It's the first place they could remember a sense of family. It's the place they brought that first boyfriend or girlfriend. It's the place they parked their first car. It holds a very special "first place" in their hearts.

Even if there is no long history, a home to the vast majority of Americans represents a sense of autonomy and control. It is not accidental in American History that people have risked their lives and fortunes to stake out something called home.

> It is your home that makes the greatest statement about your belief in the future.

It is in your home that you can wander about eating, drinking, thinking, watching and reading what you will. It is in your home that you can think the thoughts and say the things that are totally yours and totally protected once you think and say them. It is your home that makes the greatest statement about your belief in the future. It's why we talk about our dream home in such idealistic terms. The dream home is the epitome of sanctuary, safety, security, and solace. Even if it isn't all those things it still represents something special to each and every one of us.

Talking with your parents about what they're going to do with their home when they leave is a lot like asking them what they're going to do if they get divorced; it's a hypothetical that everyone should acknowledge but not spend a long time indulging.

The D.O.S. Conversation* is a perfect way to begin the conversation about the home. The R-Factor Question* could be modified to sound something like this:

"If we were sitting here three years from now and looking back to this day and you had made some decisions about your house in relation to your long-term care, what has to happen in those decisions for you to feel good about them?"

What this question does is to ask them to consider what they would decide about the house if they had made that decision in the context of their long-term care. You aren't actually asking them to decide. What you are asking them to do is to imagine a future where they are not in the house and to describe for you what has happened along the way for them to feel good about the hypothetical decision to leave. It is important that they **(1) formulate a vision of what that looks like and (2) that they trust you enough to discuss it with you.**

If you listen carefully they may reveal to you the triggering events that would make them reconsider living in their home. Most folks deal with really serious topics by a bit of humor. It relieves the tension and allows them to ease into the really important things they're considering. If your parents are anything like mine, you might hear things like:

"I'm never leaving here; they'll have to carry me out."

"I could never organize this place enough to be able to leave it."

"Who would buy this old place anyway?"

But also, you may hear them begin to articulate the things that are making them reflect upon that even now. Things like:

"Well, we really need to do some things before we could even begin to put it on the market."

"The steps are really getting to be a little bit more than they used to."

"I'm noticing that it takes a couple of days to get the yard work done now instead of one."

The D.O.S. Conversation* flows quite nicely here. You're asking them to consider what they are concerned about with this decision, what they're excited about and what strengths or advantages if any, that they're bringing to this situation. Here's how The D.O.S. Conversation might flow after they've answered the question about the house:

"If we were looking forward over the next 3 years and you were awake at 2:00 in the morning thinking about this house, what is it that would make you concerned, worried, or fearful about all of this?"

The answers to this are as varied as the number of people and the number of houses. Typically, what people are afraid of is losing control over some aspect of this decision or an actual financial loss (that they can't afford) should they sell the house. Remember that dangers here are always about the fear of loss or the actual experience of loss. Here are some common fears about the house:

- There are too many repairs to be done.
- The market is soft, we'd lose too much now.

- We would owe too much in taxes.
- This house is too old to sell.
- No one but old folks would want this house.
- We don't want people traipsing through looking at our stuff.
- Where would we go, everything is so expensive.
- After commissions, taxes, and the bank, we wouldn't have any money at all.
- Where would we live, there's nothing available.

Remember that the fears are real. Do not minimize what they fear about the house. It's their fear, their reality about the house. Your role is to help them transform that fear into a set of decisions that lets them think, communicate, and act on a plan about those fears. The plans are potentially as unlimited and creative as you can imagine.

The next question is the opportunity question. It's designed to help them discuss if there is anything to be excited about on this decision.

"If we were looking forward over the next 3 years, and you were up at 2:00 in the morning thinking about this house, what would you be excited about?"

Remember that opportunity is always about the possibility for gain. So, what is it about the house decision that could cause any set of parents to be excited? I think you may be surprised at the answers.

- We can finally get all the money we've had tied up in this house out and do some fun things.

- I'm really looking forward to a fall where I don't
  have to clean gutters and rake leaves.
- It'll give us a chance to clean things out the way
  we've been talking about.

The excitements about this are just that, their excitements.
Remember that this house decision is about them and their
relationship to the house, not about you and your relationship
with the house. They may ask you for your
opinion. Be sure and tell them that you will
give it to them only after they share their
opinion with you.

Remember that this house decision is about them and their relationship to the house...

After you discover with them what they
are afraid of and what they are excited
about, it's time for them to discover what
strengths or advantages they have in
helping them to minimize their fears and
maximize their excitement.

So, you might say:

**"Now that we know what you're afraid of and what you're
excited about concerning this house, let me ask you about the
strengths or advantages that you bring to this situation to
really help minimize your fears and maximize your
excitement."**

Your parents may need some help with this one, but you'll
probably run across some answers like these:

- Well, we are in good health and we can really live
  here without worry until we decide.

- We've had a lot of work done recently to bring the place up to speed and it really looks good.
- We have built up a lot of profit and could really go buy anything we wanted to.
- We've been thinking about this for a long time and now is as good a time as any to make this decision.

In the Tools section of *The Parent Care Solution* there is a whole checklist of things that your parents can work on together or with you to maximize their opportunities and minimize the loss in all the decisions surrounding the house.

There is a statement made when you decide to leave your home whether it's uttered aloud or not. The statement is really one to yourself and to the world that you are acknowledging the transition you must make, that you are acknowledging the part of the human experience cycle that you are leaving and the one you are entering. This transition like all transitions has an interesting balance of sadness and joy. If at all possible in this conversation help your parents celebrate the joys of the life that they are leaving and look forward to the new one they are creating no matter what the circumstances. It's one thing to acknowledge that things are sad, it's quite another to indulge it for a lifetime.

There is a temptation during times like these to make an over generalized statement that things are over. Things aren't over; they're just different.

THE HOUSE CONVERSATION

R-Factor Question*	If we were sitting here in this same time and place a year from now and looking back, what decisions about your house do you have to have made to feel **good** about your progress?
D.	If we were to look forward over the next year at the house decision, what is it that you find **fearful** about making this decision?
O.	If we were to look forward over the next year at the house decision what is it that you find **exciting** about making this decision?
S.	What is it, in the form of strengths or advantages that you bring to this decision to help **minimize** the things that concern you and **maximize** the things that excite you?

THE HOUSE CONVERSATION
Answers

D. DANGERS
- Can't sell
- Won't sell
- Too little money
- Too many repairs
- Bad market
- Tight credit
- Bad local borrowing
- Have no place to go
- Expensive future repairs
- Expensive current repairs
- Don't maximize all the value

O. OPPORTUNITIES
- Free-up cash
- Remove maintenance responsibilities
- Eliminate future repairs
- Organize belongings
- Have greater support
- Hedge against loss by selling
- Remove debt obligation

S. STRENGTHS
- Great house
- Great location
- No debt
- Willing to move
- Maximized existing potential
- Shift future maintenance to someone

CHAPTER SIX

The Property Conversation

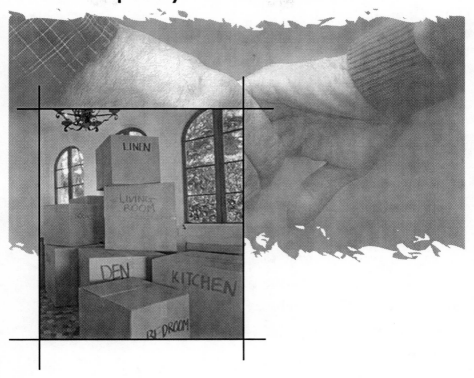

There's an interesting parallel between personal property and sibling relationships. Both of them start out new and shiny and fresh. Over time there's some wearing and little nicks and cuts that appear. As the years pass, cracks appear from place to place and the glue that once held everything together begins to yellow and harden and pull away from the very thing it was designed to bring together. If enough stress is placed at just the right time, say on a table top or a chair leg it may splinter, or crack. Usually at the most inappropriate moment the entire piece crumbles from the weight it has endured all the years. Fate and time and circumstance combine to create the perfect storm for relationship collapse.

Sibling relationships that have endured for years may be torn asunder by a picture, a hope chest, a wedding ring. Brothers and sisters who have never spoken an unkind word are suddenly across from each other with strained voices and glaring gazes. Years of thinking about the day when the "thing" of mom and dad's becomes yours erupt in swells of possessive emotion.

Sound overly dramatic? Sound unrealistic? As a lawyer, financial advisor, and gatekeeper for families, I have seen, been part of, and experienced the scenarios above. Most of the confusion, if not all of the turmoil in the scenes above could have been avoided with clear concise, and calm conversations about who should have what, when and if for any sum, how much.

While my tendency is to substitute simple language for heavy psychoanalytic theory nonetheless, there are some interesting things going on here. Personal property has for centuries been a symbol of power, influence, and status. From the early Pharaohs to the highest of high-ranking military officers, objects of personal property were included as symbols of power in this existence and as devices for protection in the world to come.

Now, you wonder, what does all that have to do with dad's watch or mother's needlework of Washington at Valley Forge?

Everything really. We sometimes need those things as human beings to stimulate or access the great memories and experiences we had with those individuals. Like our own memory box, we hold them and touch them and feel their power to bring back, if just a moment, the memory of the one that has departed.

The Parent Care Property Conversation strives to avoid all of the turmoil above and to replace it with a conversation that can run the gamut from conflict to collaboration. In this section of *The Parent Care Solution* we have tried to provide both an understanding and modeling of how conflict may be perceived, engaged, and resolved for different people with different styles under various circumstances. I am not naive enough to think that every conversation in *The Parent Care Solution* is entered into by walking across a daisy carpet smelling lilacs, but neither do they have to be the battle scenes in Braveheart.

The Parent Care Property Conversation uses The D.O.S. Conversation* but it also asks both parents and children to consider asking for what they want and being able to say it without tears of anguish getting in the way of something important. Will there be situations where the parties want the same thing? Yes. Will there be situations where you arrive at a stalemate with neither side wanting to give in? Yes. That's quite possible. How is that you say? It is possible because people fight over the silliest things including the needlework. Hopefully the gene pools in your sibling relationships are at a more advanced level.

The Parent Care Property Conversation begins with this:

"If we were all sitting here 3 years from now and looking

back to this same time and place what decisions will you have had to make about your personal possessions for you to feel comfortable with those decisions?"

Notice we didn't say, "Who will you have given the chair to, me or Bill?" What we're looking for here is their view of the future concerning what they want to do with all their stuff. The important thing here is not to begin a Big 4 audit conversation. You're really listening for some decisions they've already made, some decisions they're considering, and some decisions that they have yet to reach conclusions on.

The next question is the Dangers Questions:

"If we were to look forward over the next year and you were to find yourself up at 2:00 in the morning and you were concerned about these types of decisions, what are the things you would be concerned about?"

Every parent with children has thought about the effect of leaving certain things to one child as apposed to another. Their greatest fear is that they create dissention among their children for the decisions they have made. The easier part for most parents is to have oblique conversations along the way and let the family attorney or executor sort it out at the reading of the will.

The excitement question may get you closer to some things that they have already resolved.

"If we were to look forward over the next year and you were to find yourself up at 2:00 in the morning and you were excited about some of these decisions, what are the things you would be excited about?" (In other words, what have you already agreed to.)

Just as every parent has issues about what they don't want to discuss about their things, every parent has things they are excited about. They may have thought of each child in a special way so that the particular object is one that they know that child would value and appreciate. They may be excited because they know their children can sort it all out as they've sorted other things out for years.

The final question in the series is about the advantages they bring to the table to help them resolve these issues of property.

"As you consider the things you are concerned about and the things you are excited about when it comes to your property, what are the advantages that you bring to this situation to help you minimize your concerns and maximize your opportunities?"

Many parties will struggle with this, but with a little prompting, they'll understand that what you're really asking them to do is to talk about the things that have worked and to minimize the things that haven't. Every parent wants to be remembered for what they created in this experience called family. Over the years it has been interesting to have my entrepreneurial clients list their family as one of the things they're the most proud of, the thing that they would not exchange for anything.

Perhaps there are personal things of such great value that

> Every parent wants to be remembered for what they created in this experience called family.

53

lawsuits should be filed and relationships broken. In the very thin air of aristocracy, perhaps all those things mean a great deal. It has always been a paradox for me that for as much of our life is spent collecting, purchasing, and exhibiting both the passageway into the world and the box in which we leave it allow for really very few accessories.

THE PROPERTY CONVERSATION

R-Factor Question*

If we were sitting here in this same time and place a year from now and looking back, what decisions about your property do you have to have made to feel **good** about your progress?

D. If we were to look forward over the next year at the property decision, what is it that you find **fearful** about making this decision?

O. If we were to look forward over the next year at the property decision, what is it that you find **exciting** about making this decision?

S. What is it, in the form of strengths or advantages that you bring to this decision to help **minimize** the things that scare you and **maximize** the things that excite you?

THE PROPERTY CONVERSATION
Answers

D. DANGERS
- Can't decide to decide
- Can't decide who should have what
- Want to hold on to everything
- Too much stuff to even begin
- Children will not be happy with my decisions
- Don't want to treat children unequally
- Don't want to make decisions now
- I'll just let children decide when I'm gone

O. OPPORTUNITIES
- Great time to inventory and clean out
- Can experience joy at giving now
- Children will enjoy these things now
- Can determine real value of things
- Can organize everything for once and all
- A great time for a garage sale

S. STRENGTHS
- Am clear about what's valuable
- Am clear about what I want to give away
- Am clear about who gets what
- Have already decided some things
- Have already given away some things
- Have been organizing for some time now
- Am prepared to make transition with property
- Understand I need to do this

CHAPTER SEVEN

The Care Conversation

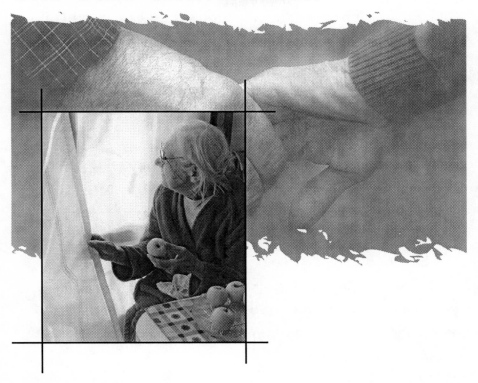

T he Care Conversation is an interesting one in that it
involves so many considerations from both a professional
standard of care that is to be delivered and also a child-parent
standard of care that may be expected. If you substitute the word
'attention' for the word 'care' the conversation becomes a bit
more manageable.

In the Tools section at the back of the book is a "Quick-
Check" checklist for The Care Conversation*. The Care
Conversation is the first conversation that involves two different
types of D.O.S. Conversations. The first D.O.S. Conversation*

is about the relationship between your parents and whomever it will be that will be providing the professional care whether it be in a retirement community, assisted living, special-care or skilled nursing facility.

The second D.O.S. Conversation is really about the type of care (translate – attention) that your parents might expect from a family member. This type of attention is really more about communication and relationship with your parents than it is about whether lotions and prescriptions are being administered properly.

The professional care conversation is concerned with what your parents see as their physical, emotional, and intellectual needs in a care community no matter what the level of entry. Those needs involve things that we call the 3M's – **Meals, Meetings,** and **Meaning**. Let me elaborate.

> The professional care conversation is concerned with what your parents see as their physical, emotional, and intellectual needs in a care community

Meals is about more than the 3 daily ones and whether they meet the RDA for a senior's system. **Meetings** is about where you can dine and whom you can dine with. In any kind of care facility meals can be fixed inside your own apartment or served to you at communal dining facilities. In many care situations, communal dining is an opportunity to develop a new set of relationships, conversations, and other connections, all of which provide **Meaning**. Fixing your meals and eating alone may be a statement about independence, but it is not about community. Conversely being forced to dine with groups of strangers each night may serve to drive one to the life of gastric solitude.

The Care Conversation here is also about the facility itself. You'll be asking your parents to describe what their new place or residence would look like at various stages of their care if they could have it just the way they wanted. You'll be asking them what they see as the potential concerns in a new living space as well as the things that excite them. You'll also discover the resources that help them bring these advantages to their best use. In the Care Facilities Checklist, you'll find a guide to provide a reasonable level of comfort about the capabilities of the facility. What you're looking for in this conversation is not a building inspection report, but rather an image of the type of surroundings that will create confidence, clarity, and connectedness for your parents. As someone who loves art, southwestern colors, space, and clutterless rooms, moving into a facility with institutionally painted walls, tile floors and indoor/outdoor carpeting would not be conducive at all to my mental health. Conversely, in the latter stages of Alzheimer's it's hard for the individual to differentiate between a luxury hotel and a closet if you could remember which one you're in… and of course you can't. Finances, proximately to family, and simple availability all go into the facilities consideration.

The most challenging, the most sensitive, the most rewarding care conversation is the one you have with your parents about their expectations of your care relationship with them. Like everything else in these conversations, care may have a multitude of meanings depending on the context.

Care may mean the actual physical day-to-day care that your parents need. It runs the gamut from waking them up with a coffee and paper, to daily medicine, diapers and doctors.

Care may also mean the emotional attention that your parents want from you at this stage of their life that they may or may not be able to articulate. Care most often hides in unveiled expectations. It, like the physical care can run along the continuum from stopping by the facility on Thanksgiving, Christmas, and their birthdays to visiting daily or merely helping with meals and interacting with the staff.

The D.O.S. Conversation* is incredibly useful here. When we were contemplating my father's care nearly six years ago, I asked him a slightly altered form of the question. His reply was typical of that generation of men who if they were aware of their inner life, couldn't articulate it well, or if they weren't aware still could not bring themselves to answer in any form. His reply to my question was a mixture of humor, sarcasm and a veiled fear of being forgotten. He replied that he hoped I would come on the Big Ones (Thanksgiving, Easter, Fourth of July, his birthday) and if I could remember it, some of the other ones. While he never described them exactly, it was clear that he was saying in his own way that he didn't want to be forgotten. He also told me to come anytime I needed money. That comment was strange in that it had been years since I had been to him for anything like that and even more strange since I had a complete power of attorney to handle his financial affairs.

Caregivers have an interesting task. Whether you've been formally trained to do this such as a nurse or doctor or therapist, or whether you were thrust into the role and learned on the job, the experience emotionally, physically, and intellectually is very much the same.

My experience with care giving is different than yours will be and yours will be different from someone else's. In fact, we can both be caring for the same person (a parent for example) and will have a totally different experience even though we may manage many of the same details.

Care giving is many things. It is a duty, an honor, a burden, and frequently a pain in the butt. It is, to borrow from Dickens, "The best of times and the worst of times." It is the feeling of limitless joy and feeling of bottomless despair. It is walking to the car remarking how well he or she was today and laughing. It is crying on the way to the car thinking that if only this could end, and they could end, there would be an end to all of the pain.

I have a theory that in old age you become more of what you've already been. Based on an abstract idea that life somehow or another accumulates, old age may be nothing more than an entire life with an exponent attached. I think if you've been happy most of your life, in old age, all things being equal you remain as happy or become more so. If you have been unhappy most of your life, the same is true. My experience in handing the financial affairs of folks over the years suggests that the same is true with their lifelong experience with money. If you have been fearful, miserly, or have struggled with money, absent a great windfall, old age brings more or less the same. If you have had a prosperous experience, had a feeling of abundance, and practiced a sort of financial benevolence, old age, absent a catastrophic occurrence is much the same.

Care giving is the same way. I am only sure of this one thing in the care giving experience; that you are the same type of caregiver that you are a person. All care giving does is provide a forum where those characteristics get revealed or magnified.

> Care giving is both an honor and a duty.

Care giving is both an honor and a duty. It is an honor in that you have volunteered or have been selected to become an attendant to what I believe is a certain nobility, that of your parents. Everyone reading this book has, however brief, experienced at one point what it has felt like to be the most important person on earth. Their feeling about this more likely than not came from parents…those people who brought you into the world, made you the world they revolved around, and who fed you, clothed you, and trained you to be a part of the bigger world. They for a while were the king and queen in a kingdom called You. It is only fitting that, in this the last stages of their reign that you should attend to them the way that nobility is attended to. Their reigns, like all reigns will come to an end far too soon.

Care giving is a duty. It is not for the faint hearted. It is not for the weak-minded. It is not for sissies... It is clearly not for sissies.

It is a duty because you must do it once you have agreed to it no matter what the circumstances. You must do it when they know you are there and you must do it when they aren't aware. You must do it when the elements are in your favor; sun, sky, and breeze and you must do it when they are not. You must do it when a thousand voices tell you in your head to skip just this one time and you must do it when everything in you tells you that you should be and want to be doing something else. It is a duty because many will start with you; brothers, sisters, friends, but only a few will choose to finish with you. Not only will you have your part of the job to do, but also you will have their part of the job, because there is no one else but you to do it and therefore you must. You must do it when you feel like it and you must do it when you don't. You must do it when you are appreciated and when you are taken for granted. You must do it when there are a thousand things you would rather be doing than this. Care giving may in the beginning and the end be an act of love, I am sure in the long middle, it is an exercise of will.

Care giving is an act of generosity and it is in that generosity the huge dangers lie. It is possible as a caregiver to deplete your stores of energy, intellect, money and time. It is possible to run out of all of these in this indeterminate time frame of benevolence you have entered. When the resources of time, money, love and dedication are gone, what rushes in is resentment, bitterness, anger, and exhaustion.

The D.O.S. Conversation* is an important one not only to

have with your parents about their expectations with you but for you to have with your expectations for your self about them. I have included a sample for each scenario for you to consider.

Since I am some place in the "middle" in my care giving experience, I cannot with any certainty tell you how I will feel in the end. The descriptions of what care giving is in the first of the chapter should at least convince you that I am no casual observer here, no mere audience member laughing on cue and crying at the sad parts, only to rise after a brief time to go and join another world. No, I am a full-fledged member of the caregiving cast. The move from audience member to cast member is interesting. The change in perspective is dramatic.

> *The Parent Care Solution* allows you to acknowledge the care situation that's required, but not to indulge it.

What I hope you see in these conversations is that I have not plunged into any state of shock nor have I indulged in the readily available tonics of denial, guilt, blame, anger, or depression. Rather, I have used all of what has happened to transform myself, to transform the situation for my father, and to transform the experience that I am having throughout this entire process. In fact, *The Parent Care Solution* is my attempt to transform not only my experience with this situation, but to enable others to transform the same experience in their lives. *The Parent Care Solution* allows you to acknowledge the care situation that's required, but not to indulge it.

The great Indian poet Rabindranath Tragore summarized this whole caregiver responsibility rather nicely when he wrote:

"I looked and thought that life was duty
I slept and dreamt that life was joy
I awoke and knew that duty was joy."

My hope is that your care giving experience is both duty and joy.

THE CARE *FACILITY* CONVERSATION

R-Factor Question*	If we were sitting here in this same time and place a year from now and looking back, what decisions about the care facility do you have to have made to feel **good** about your progress?
D.	If we were to look forward over the next year at the care facility decision, what is it that you find **fearful** about making this decision?
O.	If we were to look forward over the next year at the care facility decision what is it that you find **exciting** about making this decision?
S.	What is it, in the form of strengths or advantages that you bring to this decision to help **minimize** the things that scare you and **maximize** the things that excite you?

THE CARE *FACILITY* CONVERSATION
Answers

D. DANGERS
- Don't know how to evaluate
- Will choose the wrong person
- Will not be happy with the person
- Can't be sure of background
- Can't monitor or supervise
- Too expensive
- Too much turnover
- Will have a stranger taking care of me
- Won't like facility
- Facility won't be like home
- Family may not support decision

O. OPPORTUNITIES
- Comfortable surroundings
- Community to join
- Central place for activities
- Increased socialization
- Balanced diet, health care
- Organized exercise, activities
- On site medical attention
- Transitional living phase possible
- Increased family control
- No home responsibilities
- Daily bills/tasks taken care of

S. STRENGTHS
- Have or can get financial resources
- Have prepared financially, emotionally for decision
- Have evaluated best possible care options
- Family is in support of idea
- Have prepared to leave my home
- Am ready for transition
- Some of my friends have already made this decision
- Have always been easily adaptable in new situations
- I understand all the consequences of my decision

THE CARE *ATTENTION* CONVERSATION

R-Factor Question*

If we were sitting here in this same time and place one year from now and looking back to today, what is it about your family's attention that you would have liked to discuss in order to feel **good** about your relationship with them?

D. If you were to look forward over the next year, what is it about the level of attention from your family that makes you **fearful**?

O. If you were to look forward over the next year, what is it about the level of attention from your family that gives you a reason to be **excited**?

S. What is it that you believe you bring to this need for attention from your family that **minimizes** your concerns and **increases** your excitement?

THE CARE *ATTENTION* CONVERSATION
Answers

D. **DANGERS**
- You will forget about me.
- You won't visit enough.
- You won't stay long when you do visit.
- We won't have anything to talk about.
- You'll come by less and less as I get older and more ill.
- You won't want to be around me when I'm sick.
- You won't bring my grandchildren
- I'll get sick and die by myself.
- You won't help me see my friends.
- I won't get to get out and about.

O. **OPPORTUNITIES**
- We can develop a new and different relationship.
- We have more time for quiet focused conversation.
- We can deepen our existing relationship.
- We can have more opportunities to share and visit.
- We can expand our topics of conversation.
- I can see my grandchildren more.
- I can share with you the story of my life on an ongoing basis.
- I won't be distracted by all the things I have to do.
- We could actually deepen and expand our relationship.

S. **STRENGTHS**
- We've always had a mutual respect for each other.
- We have a long history of making a best effort with each other.
- We have always prepared for this time.
- We started some of these conversations long ago.
- I am really open to a deeper more connected relationship.
- I have always known that you would stay connected to me in my older years.
- We have a good connection through the grandchildren that will strengthen our desire to come together.

CHAPTER EIGHT

The Legacy Conversation

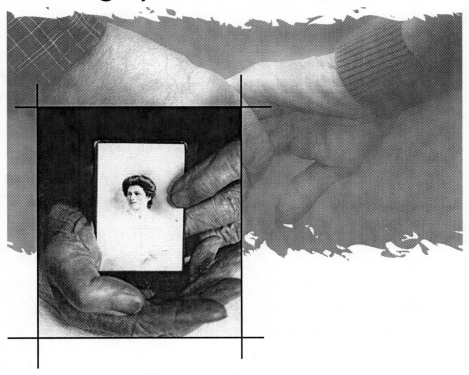

The **Legacy Conversation** is about being remembered. The least of us wants to be remembered. The most important of us wants to be remembered. All of us want to be remembered in some way or another whether we admit it or not. The Legacy Conversation is admitting you want to be remembered but it is also telling people how you want to be remembered.

There are numerous ways in the 21st century to document a memory. Some are digital like snapshots and video. Some are on plain paper, like obituaries. Others take their form in marble, bronze, and stone at gravesites or mausoleums. Whatever the form you choose, they all have in common a structure of memory.

The D.O.S. Conversation* is a fascinating way to approach the subject of legacy because it allows the person you've asked to really describe how they would like to be remembered but also to share how they would not like to be thought of (the dangers) how they would like to be thought of (the excitements) and all the accomplishments (advantages) they brought to their life and others' as they moved through their journey. It is often said that we rarely remember what a man or woman had when they passed, but we always remember what they were. What they were is the combination of all the things that created the context in which they lived and moved about.

I think that parents and children have a common thread that unites them in these conversations. Parents want to know that they have truly made a contribution to their children, their friends, and their community. Their children, in the end, want to know that they have acted nobly within that contribution. Each is looking for the other to acknowledge their contributions.

> Parents want to know that they have truly made a contribution to their children, their friends, and their community.

When I was thinking about how to talk with my father about this legacy with me and with the world I struggled a lot. How do you have a conversation like this without making it feel like a last goodbye speech or some sort of awkward soliloquy of things that should've been said, but weren't, of things that could've been accomplished but weren't, of things that were supposed to happen but didn't.

The purpose of this conversation is not to create a checklist, add up the score and then pronounce the life valuable or not. It is really to create confidence between you and your parents about the past of your relationship, the present of your relationship, and yes, the future of your relationship.

The best definition of confidence I have ever experienced is the definition I learned from my friend, Dan Sullivan.

"Confidence is the ability to transform fear into very focused thinking, communication, and action – with the result that weaknesses become strengths, obstacles become innovations, and setbacks become breakthroughs."

Why focus on confidence in a conversation between parents and child at this point in everyone's life? What does confidence have to do with anything here? Why focus on confidence when there are literally dozens of other things to focus and talk about?

Here's why. Your primary role, indeed the most important role that you have as a caregiver and as a child is to provide confidence to your parents in this situation. Confidence as you will soon see is a fairly integrated set of emotional, intellectual and physical actions that can literally transform the experience of your parents at this point in their life as well as your own experience in this situation.

Let's look at the definition of confidence. Confidence is first of all, the ability to transform *fear*. Fear about what?

- **About not doing well enough in the past**
- **About not being able to take care of themselves in the present**
- **About being a burden in the future**

All parents share a fear that they could've done more of everything "if only". If only I would have had more _____. (You fill in the blank: money, time, energy, love, caring, togetherness, relationship, education, promotion, spare change, money for summer camp) then everything would've been _____ (the real word they want to put here is 'perfect', but they'll substitute ok, better, different).

You can have the same fears about your relationships with them. Stay on this "disease of more" and "if only" path and you will all end up in state hospitals drinking Prozac slurpies.

Your role in this conversation is to help them transform that fear into:

- **Very focused thinking about the past, the present, and the future**
- **Very focused action about the past, the present and the future**
- **Very focused communication about the past, the present and the future**

You do this focused thinking thing so that you can help them see and understand that what they perceive as:

- **Weaknesses** in their past, present and future are really opportunities for innovative ideas, and thinking relationships to promote and develop their ideas of progress for themselves and with you.

- **Obstacles** in their past, present, and future are really strengths they developed as they continued to make progress in their lives for themselves and with you.

- **Setbacks** in their past, present and future were really and are now and in the future opportunities for breakthroughs in growth, development, relationship and thinking for themselves and with you.

A legacy is in part about reconstructing the past so that it makes sense, organizing the present to transcend that past, and designing a future that honors and integrates all that has gone before. A legacy is really an exercise in identifying the progress in a human life.

I will tell you that I do not believe that there is one single life on the planet that has not made some type of progress for some amount of time in its existence. Being born is the first step on the progress path. Fifty million sperm after one egg and you won out. Give me a break. Just getting born should win the lifetime achievement award. Learning to speak, write, learn, relate, provide for oneself, give to others. All these are huge progress milestones.

Your job with your parents in this conversation is to get them to reflect on their past in a way that maximizes their progress and minimizes their disappointment and setbacks. Remember that all history in the end is revisionist. We all reconstruct the past to best suit our way of remembering. Now, I'm not saying that you lie about your past, that you fabricate things to embellish your story. For example, you don't let your parents say they knew Orville and Wilbur Wright in order to justify their love for flying. That's an exercise in delusionary thinking not historical reflection. What I am saying is that you have a perfect right to interpret the events, people, and past in a way that allows you to celebrate some sort of progress. If the psychological community can make billions bringing up all the stuff in your past that didn't work and using it to explain your present, why can't you just tweak that a bit and use it for all the reasons to explain your progress and the viability of your future?

Legacy is about confident conversation because there is so much fear to transform. So, what you are charged with doing is bringing confidence to the planning for your parents' care, for the implementation of these decisions and for the successful navigation of the waters that lie ahead. From the moment you start interacting with your parents about their long-term care you will have a mission, a focus, and a plan of confidence.

> Legacy is about confident conversation because there is so much fear to transform.

All that is great you say, but where does my confidence come from in order to help them with theirs? After all, I'm the one making the arrangements, the trips, and the visits to provide them with all this confidence, where does mine come from? And even more important, how do I continually replenish the supply?

Not easy questions. In fact they are great, relative, and meaningful questions. How do you keep your confidence in full supply in this situation?

It is tempting here to launch into the trite. Get plenty of rest, or drink lots of liquids, and take your vitamins. The truth is you need to do those things to not only stay confident, but to stay healthy. Here's how you stay confident:

Be Grateful. That's right, pure and simple gratitude. Gratitude from the Koran. Gratitude from the New Testament. Gratitude from the sayings of Buddha. Gratitude from the Navaho. Whatever the source, gratitude.

Gratitude allows you to stay confident in that being grateful simply restores your energy. I'm not saying that you wander about pie-eyed, sniffing incense and sprinkling lilac water on gangrene. That's not being grateful. That's being silly.

Gratitude is about reflecting positively about all those things that happened in the past, all those things that are happening now, and all those things that are likely to happen in the future. Being grateful allows you to experience all those things for what they were, for what they are, and for what they will be in contributing to your growth. All of this parent care stuff is really just about growth and development. At the risk of sounding like a week of Yanni concerts, there's huge opportunity for growth in this situation with your parents. Well, let me rephrase that…there is growth or there isn't. It's really that simple.

The reason The D.O.S. Conversation* works so well here is that the question really lets your parents talk about how they would like to be remembered. It lets them talk about what scares them in that memory, what excites them in that memory, what strengths they would like to be remembered for.

The D.O.S. Conversation* took place with my father really 3 years ago when he could still make the words in his head come together as sentences and say them. All Alzheimer's patients have moments that are clearer than others. Due to some unknown combination of light, energy, nutrition, and circulation the brain, from moment to moment, rights itself and there are occasions of clarity that are wonderful.

I was visiting with my father when one of those moments occurred. I saw from his posture, his focus, his speech that he was back, not like he used to be, but enough to have a conversation.

So, I asked him the question in a way that he would be able to respond.

"Dad, if we were sitting here a year from now, and looking back, what is that you would want to have said about you and your life so that you feel good about having lived?"

I waited for the answer. After what seemed to me to be an ice age of silence, he said:

"I would like people to say that I was honest, that I cared for my family, and that I always tried to do what was right. And another thing. That you could always depend on me."

I asked. "Which one of those things is most important to you?"

He replied: "That I took care of my family."

I asked him if there were some fears about being remembered in a certain way. He said that there were times when he had to be tough to get his job done, and that sometimes he was hard on us, and that he didn't want to be remembered as just a tough, hard guy but as a guy who was tough and hard at times because that's what he thought he had to be but that really wasn't who he was.

We mulled over that together and then I asked him what he was most excited about in his life.

He said that to see us (his children) grow up and live our lives was a real happy thing for him. He said that he had loved our mom and that he had missed her every day since she had passed in 1991.

I told him that I thought that he had created a remarkable life for himself and his family and that the very hard, poverty-stricken West Virginia background may have been the inspiration for him to do so well. So, I asked what he thought his strengths were that helped him in his life with all its challenges and opportunities.

He looked at me, puzzled, as if no one had ever asked him to talk about himself like this before. He said, "You mean you want me to tell you what I'm good at?" I said, "Yes, why don't you tell me what it is you're good at."

For the next half hour he talked about how growing up really poor had helped him to appreciate every little thing. He told me how he used to ride his bicycle to school without gloves so he had to learn how to ride without any hands so that he could keep his hands in his pockets. He could ride 5 miles like that before it was over.

He talked about how his family had been the reason he came back alive from the war. He was in WWII on the U.S.S. North Carolina during the Battle of Pelelieu in the South Pacific. He said as he saw the wounded and dying being brought from shore that he felt like dying, just giving up. He said that war was one of the most horrible things he had ever experienced and that it changed him forever.

He paused and then shared that he thought growing up on a farm had given him respect for hard work, and the value of doing a days work for a days pay, and that always earning his money had been a real source of pride for him. He told me about getting the same toy wagon two years in a row at Christmas. The first year it was new. The second year it was repainted because it was the Depression and there was no money.

As I was listening it occurred to me that what we all want in some way is for our story to get heard and remembered, and told again from time-to-time. It is in our story that we live forever. Immortality has but one form, be it story, or legend, or myth. The philosopher Erickson wrote, "I am what survives me". In the end we all are what survives us.

> As I listened to him, I realized how much without ever realizing it, he had been an inspiration to me.

I had not grasped the full power of The D.O.S. Conversation* until that evening with my father. It was The D.O.S. Conversation that was allowing him to open up, to say what he wanted to about him, because for the first time in his life the questions really were about him. He didn't have to tell a story about himself every now and then for effect or to emphasize a point, the whole story was really about him in this conversation.

As I listened to him, I realized how much without ever realizing it, he had been an inspiration to me. How much I had adopted his drive, his energy, and his determination in my own life. Even now, he was that source of inspiration …in my business, this writing, the books, everything.

We never talked like that again. Over the next few months the disease that had upset his life began to take control and gradually our conversation dwindled to smiles and the trite "Hi, good to see you" that Alzheimer's barely makes possible.

The Legacy Conversation via The D.O.S. Conversation* is a great transformer for all parties. In this instance it brought a sense of connectedness, closure, and communication that would've seemed unimaginable a few years ago. It allowed for connection. It allowed for communication. It allowed for conversation. More importantly, it allowed a story to be created; his story, that will be in our hearts, on our minds, and told around the campfire for generations to come.

After all, there's really nothing like a good story.

THE LEGACY CONVERSATION

R-Factor Question*
If we were sitting here in this same time and place one year from now and looking back, what is it that you would like to be remembered for to feel **good** about your life thus far?

D. If we were to look forward over the next year at the memories of your life, what is it that you find **fearful** about those memories?

O. If we were to look forward over the next year at the memories of your life what is it that you would find **exciting** about your personal legacy?

S. What is it, in the form of strengths or advantages that you bring to this reflection of your life to help **minimize** the things that scare you and **maximize** the things that excite you?

THE LEGACY CONVERSATION
Answers

D. DANGERS
- It won't be important to anyone that I was alive
- I will be remembered in the wrong way
- I will only be remembered for what I didn't do
- Will have lost relationship opportunities
- People will focus on my faults
- Will never get to say what I want to say
- I will be forgotten

O. OPPORTUNITIES
- Can say what I want to people I care about
- Can communicate what was important to me
- Can communicate my philosophy, values,
- Can shape "my story" for future generations
- Can build on great family history
- Can be remembered for the things that I thought were important for me.

S. STRENGTHS
- Has always been easy to talk to family
- Children have been willing to listen
- Family wants to have this conversation
- Have been thinking about this for some time
- Am clear about how I want to be remembered
- Have a long history of great family communication

CHAPTER NINE

27 Reasons

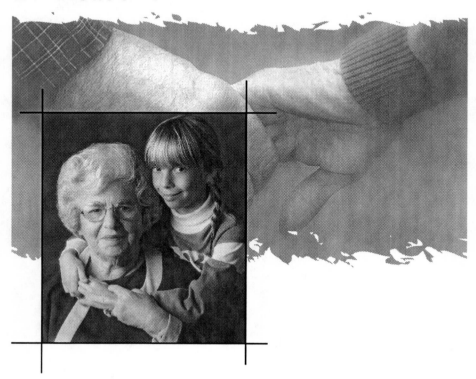

The twenty-seven reasons is a not so subtle attempt to strip away all the excuses the Boomer Generation may have for not engaging with their parents on the topic of long-term care. The purpose of the 27 reasons is to come to grips with the realities of that long-term care relationship and to decide if and how you want to interact with your parents on this issue. While the 27 reasons were written from the Boomer's perspective, it does not take a great deal of word replacement to know that the parents can have these same reasons for not talking to their children.

The 27 reasons that follow are not an attempt to anger you,

to frustrate you, or to depress you. The reasons are to stimulate you to take action or not in this very important relationship area. My hope is that in the 27 reasons you will find one of each in terms of irritation, frustration, and depression. My hope is that you find many more to stimulate you.

REASON #1: I have never talked to my parents about anything, much less their money, their health or their care.

The Parent Care Conversation is not about you; it's about your parents and the type of support, if any that they want as they approach this time in their life. The D.O.S. Conversation* if followed correctly opens up a conversation where your parents talk about their fears, their opportunities and their strengths. This is a conversation for them about their future. If they answer the questions in the D.O.S. Conversation* they will by default reveal to you the picture of their future as well as revealing whether they are comfortable enough to have a conversation with you about that future. If they will not answer these questions with you or for themselves, you have much more to be concerned with in the long term than whether they can talk with you.

> This is a conversation for them about their future.

REASON #2: My parents have things everywhere. Even they aren't sure where everything is. How do I design a plan when I can't find everything?

Unless you're attached to parents who are living on a respirator, you have just described the situation that roughly 80% of the Baby Boom Generation will find themselves. *The Parent Care Solution* doesn't promise that getting organized will be easy, just that it will be possible. The financial tools are designed to work off the barest of information sources. Start with name, address, and phone number and then move to more complicated questions. And, do it over a period of time where you and your parents are not completely stressed out.

We are not saying that getting this information will be easy, painless or free of stress and difficulty. We are saying that there are two times when you can do this: Now, while everyone is thinking clearly and can co-operate in piecing all this together, or later when you're trying to locate bank accounts, brokerage statements, wills and trusts at the same time you're trying to get them admitted to Pleasant Meadows.

Be a big person here. Take charge. Provide direction. Provide leadership. If after you tried to do this to no avail, resign yourself to the inevitable, dump the guilt and worry and try to go on about your life.

REASON #3: My parents say they've already done this with their _____ (fill in the blank with attorney, CPA, banker, broker, insurance agent, family friend, priest, rabbi, or gardener) and they don't need to do it again.

Well, maybe they have and maybe they haven't. I'm pretty clear they haven't done it with the simplicity, connectedness and thoroughness that we've outlined in this book. If they have, then they would be the first I've seen in 20+ years.

Most parents have completed pieces of the Solution. They may have purchased a long-term care policy or life insurance program. They may have executed wills or trust agreements. They may have designated health care powers and decided who the mantle clock goes to. Find out what they've done and what else needs to be done. See if you can get them to share what is already in place and make them aware of what else is necessary. They either will be open to this or they won't. Explain to them that you will not be able to be fully supportive and helpful to them if you don't know what they've done. Share with them that without knowing what has already been accomplished; you may waste precious hours and valuable resources duplicating efforts.

REASON #4: My parents are very private about their money and it was a taboo subject in our life growing up. How do I get them to open up?

It has been fascinating to me over the past 20 years how clients in our business will discuss their vacations, children, health ailments, job insecurities, and religious beliefs with family members or spouses but will not, except under penalty of death, reveal the fact they have $2,700 in a savings account somewhere.

Depression born or post-depression born children have grown up with fears concerning money that have fundamentally kept psychotherapists fully employed over the last century and savings accounts at national banks filled to overflowing with cash. I am not educated nor intuitively gifted enough to dive off that high board of conversation nor do believe there is any water to be found.

The Parent Care Solution treats money as a tool for designing a certain structure. It doesn't make judgments about whether the tools are good, bad, enough, or too little. It just uses what is there to build what it can. Try to shift the conversation from money as a secret, taboo thing indicative of power, prestige, status or the lack thereof, to something more where you think of it like a screwdriver, or chisel, or saw. When you don't have the right tools to do a job, you fundamentally face three decisions:

1. Whether you buy, borrow, or rent someone else's tools

2. Whether you choose another tool to accomplish the project or

3. Whether you just shut the project down and put it on hold.

> The Parent Care Solution treats money as a tool for designing a certain structure.

What you have to understand is that in this project called parent care, you have to talk about the money at a point or things don't happen.

Try driving up to Pleasant Acres and telling the admissions director that your parents have everything filled out but they're just uncomfortable with talking about the money. I think the reality is that they will immediately enter into the "sleep in the parking lot experience".

REASON #5: My parents and I have never been close, have

never been able to talk about anything, and rarely see or talk with each other. What do I do?

Maybe nothing. Maybe this can't work for you or them. Maybe you just decide to drop in one day at the old family home and they aren't there. In fact, maybe a new family has moved in and they didn't even meet your parents at the closing. Maybe none of this stuff is interesting enough, is important enough, is thought provoking enough to get the phone lines going between you and them. Maybe it isn't, won't, and never will be possible to have this conversation about this thing with them. Maybe it just doesn't work.

But, if it could, do you think you'd like to find out now rather than later. Both parents and children wish at some point they had a better past as far as their relationship is concerned. The better past stuff is for my friends in the counseling business. I'm pretty clear that the best chance I've got is to design a better future for them with me. If we can do that or at least begin that we have a lot to talk about going forward.

If you could talk to them and they could talk to you what would you say and when would you say it?

REASON #6: I can't do this by myself and I'm afraid of the potential conflict. What do I do?

Here's a better question. If you don't, who will? If you begin this conversation and someone else wants to be a part of it, let them or not. If they don't want to, you will never hear from them. Remember at some point in your parents' evaluation someone will have to help make decisions, or clean up messes from decisions that weren't made. Don't expect this Parent Care Conversation to be conflict free. It won't be. Why? Because it's just not that kind of planet.

REASON #7: I grew up in a very close, communicating family and I know everyone will want to be involved or at a minimum level, informed about what's going on. How do we decide who is in control?

Great question! Here's a thought. Why not let everyone be in control of their own D.O.S. Conversation* about this situation and you just be in charge of making sure that everyone's voice is heard. As far as being in control is concerned, why don't you (1) get yourself elected by the family to be in charge or (2) form a family executive committee to share decision making, responsibility, and accountability.

Again, do not look for the perfect solution: you know, the one where everyone is happy, where everyone gets everything they want. It's just not likely to happen. Instead, why don't you focus on the progress you can make together towards a solution and not try for a perfect solution? My friend Dan Sullivan at The Strategic Coach has developed a tool called "The 80% Solution" in his

"Always Increase Your Confidence" series. Try for an 80% solution where everyone's concerns are met if possible.

You actually have a terrific set of circumstances and relationships to design a very effective Parent Care Solution no matter what your situation if you'll just focus on the 80%.

REASON #8: My parents and I have lots of unresolved issues that continue to hinder our ability to talk and communicate with each other. How do we get past these to be able to talk?

At the risk of simultaneously displaying my relationship or emotional I.Q. skill deficits and offending at least half the free world's psychiatric community I would just tell you to do one thing: Get past it. Build a bridge; get over it. If it's easy, do it easy, if it's hard, do it hard. Just get it done. Get out of the "you never loved me – I didn't get a wagon- you liked Suzy better" psychobabble swamp. Realize that some things can be fixed. Some can't. Talk about what you can redesign not what you can't. Talk about the future, not the past. All the energy and hope is in the future, not in the past. Create the future. Don't rebuild the past. Your best efforts in the past will only get up to zero in the relationship rehab business. You can build a completely new structure by focusing on the future. There is no scientific evidence, no empirical studies, and no best evidence files to suggest that a thorough analysis of the past gives you a better future. Here's what gives you a better future: A better future.

Focus on the privilege, the challenges, the honor, perhaps

even the duty of helping your parents at this junction of their life. My experience has been that most issues disappear into the thin air they belong once the adult diapers go on and the respirator is attached.

REASON #9: I have my own life, my own family, my own responsibilities to take care of and I just can't do this.

Okay, then don't.

REASON #10: I just can't deal with the pain and the hurt of what will come from talking about the end of life for my parents.

Well, aren't you special. Perhaps the rest of your life, including the end of it, will be spared any undue stress, or agony, or pain. Perhaps you just golf or play tennis forever in a place where the grass is always green, the sky is always blue, and children and dogs clean up after themselves. Perhaps you just move to Lake Woebegone now.

What about growing up and sucking it up. What about realizing that this isn't about you and your hurt but about them and their care. What about stepping into a role of leadership, relationship, and creativity that brings confidence to this situation. What about being that person that deep down your parents hoped you would become when they invested all the time, energy, money, and love in creating you? What about using this as an opportunity to grow and develop your reserves of character, strength, and integrity.

What about doing anything but whining?

REASON #11: I have never been good with money and would be afraid to advise my parents about what to do or to be responsible for all of the decisions.

John Wayne and John Rambo are the only two characters that did everything alone. The rest of us mortals need some help.

The Parent Care Solution has been designed to let you work with your family's group of advisors as the

> John Wayne and John Rambo are the only two characters that did everything alone.

facilitators to utilize their years of relationship, wisdom, and experience to maximize your parent's situation. The conversations, forms, and information are all relatively easy to use.

Alternately, we have created the training for a new type of professional: a Parent Care Specialist™. The Parent Care Specialist has received specific training not only in The D.O.S. Conversation*, but also in the various tax, legal, financial, and facilities care issues to help act as the facilitator if you choose not to. The Parent Care Specialist is compensated for their wisdom and experience in assisting you in designing the appropriate strategy regardless of whether you purchase financial, legal, or tax products through them. You may of course decide to do that through a separate written agreement concerning those pieces of support with folks who are trained, licensed and regulated to provide that support.

REASON #12: Even if I could talk to my parents, how do I know whom to trust with all the decisions that have to be made?

In the financial area of life, the issue of trust really comes down to a fear of losing money. The fear of losing money is usually turned into a reality of losing money by working with or purchasing things through people who will be paid whether their solution works or not.

The Parent Care Specialist is a new professional who has been specifically trained to have The D.O.S. Conversation*, gather the necessary financial, legal, and tax information concerning your parents' affairs and then to design a strategy for their care capable of being implemented by you with your family's advisees or by you with the Parent Care Specialist and your family's advisees. If your family does not have a relationship with certain necessary advisees, the Parent Care Specialist can recommend advisors to work with you in teamwork.

The Parent Care Specialist is paid a fee for designing the Solution for your parents and is obligated to disclose any additional compensation that is received from any sources. The law requires that any professional be appropriately licensed to receive compensation directly, or indirectly in certain fields like financial planning, law, accounting, insurance, or investment advisory work. The Parent Care Specialist will not only disclose their capabilities in those areas, they will assist you, if asked, in determining the current standing of other professionals you may choose to work with.

REASON #13: I feel like I've already done a lot of the things you talk about. Why do I need to have a 'solution' designed, much less pay for it?

Well, you may have it all done and you may not. I don't know your specific situation and can't comment on whether what you've done will work for you or not.

What I do know is that *The Parent Care Solution* has been designed to provide a comprehensive, integrated strategy capable of being implemented by you and your advisors with the help of a Parent Care Specialist. It provides through its structure a network of deep support for participants. Through a variety of professional services and products designed to collaborate and not compete with The D.O.S. Conversation* of the family situation. *The Parent Care Solution* becomes a transformative process for children and their partners, which turns fears, sadness, and resentments into conversation, restoration and collaboration.

REASON #14: My parents are already in a care facility. How can *The Parent Care Solution* help them now?

It may not be able to at all. It may be that your parents made many of the important decisions prior to entering the facility and everything is well taken care of.

Our experience has been that even though parents are in a facility many of the day-to-day care issues are not being maintained to provide the best experience for parents. In addition, many parents have not made the necessary financial or legal decisions to fully protect themselves and preserve their property, privacy and person from the complicated consequences associated with aging.

The Parent Care Solution can be entered into by first using The D.O.S. Conversation* no matter what they current situation of your parents. The D.O.S. Conversation has been designed to elicit information from your parents as their situation continues to evolve and change.

REASON #15: I don't have the training or the background to discuss all these things with my parents.

This process has been designed to work in partnership with a Parent Care Specialist who does have the training, background, and experience to discuss the more technical issues of parent care.

The D.O.S. Conversation* just takes a little bit of practice to be comfortable with and is an incredibly effective tool to begin a conversation with the parents.

The background you have that is really important is the one of years of being in relationship with your parents. Presumably you are interested in *The Parent Care Solution* because you have a genuine concern for the long-term care and well being of your parents. A past history of caring and relationship is a huge advantage in beginning the conversation about your future relationship.

REASON #16: I don't see how I can afford to pay for a plan about my parents care when I can't even pay for the care

that they will need.

The Parent Care Solution has been designed to require a fraction of the total long-term care costs in the beginning to design the plan. Our experience over the years has been that folks without a plan very often make ill-advised and very expensive decisions because of not having a plan. Since there is not a set fee that a Parent Care Specialist has to charge it may be that your specialist would be flexible in terms of compensation for designing a plan for you if there were some sort of commitment of a long-term professional relationship or other ways of compensation.

> ...folks without a plan very often make ill-advised and very expensive decisions because of not having a plan.

The benefits of having a plan vs. not having a plan are really too numerous to mention. Fate, time, and circumstance have a way of creating demands on us when our energies and resources are less than at maximum capacity. By having a plan you can anticipate all but the most esoteric and unforeseen circumstances. While it is clear that all plans change once the thing you planned for begins; it is also clear that without a plan every unplanned beginning brings about a very unpredictable result.

Planning can begin with The D.O.S. Conversation* and progress as your capabilities and resources allow. Whatever you can do, begin it.

REASON #17: I have already organized all my parents'

assets, reviewed their estate plan, updated their insurance, and everything else from a financial planning standpoint that I think is necessary. What else is there to do?

Maybe nothing: but then again, maybe lots of things. The technicalities of Medicare planning, facility assessment, and caregiver selection just to name a few, all have traps for the unwary.

Even though the number of resources to do your own financial planning has multiplied over the years, the number of people who have actually availed themselves of those resources hasn't multiplied proportionately.

Even if you believe you have done a complete and thorough job in the financial area, it would be a good idea to consult with someone to reaffirm the correctness and sufficiency of these decisions. Whether you select a certified financial planner, a chartered life underwriter, CPA, attorney, or registered investment advisor, or Parent Care Specialist team with someone whose years of wisdom and experience can team with your specific preparations to create a complete result.

REASON #18: I just don't see a way to get all my siblings together to reach a consensus on what to do. Our family dynamics are not exactly normal.

The longer I'm in the world of families, the more I realize that not-the-norm is the norm. No one said getting any group together past high school graduation would be easy, much less a group of brothers and sisters.

Here are some things to try. (1) Send an email, fax, Federal Express, smoke signal or runner (however you communicate) to your siblings asking any of them if they are interested in discussing the long-term care concerns of your parents. Then work with the ones who respond using The D.O.S. Conversation* for them concerning this issue. Once you have every family members' concerns, then you can create a family D.O.S. (2) Once you have the family D.O.S. choose a key group (some number under 50) to approach your parents to (a) share your D.O.S. with them and (b) understand their D.O.S.

Will this work absolutely every time in every situation? No, it's just not that kind of planet. Will it work if you don't try it? Clearly NOT. Will it work if you try it…sometimes it will, sometimes it won't. Groups of people exhibit strange behaviors. One year a group elects a king, the next year the same group hangs him.

Just begin. Let the process unfold as it will. Once you get beyond 3 variables in any situation the average human losses the ability to conceptualize the outcome. Just have the conversation.

REASON #19: In your Parent Care Cost Recovery System you advocate insuring the lives of parents with children as beneficiaries. Isn't that kind of morbid; like profiting from your parents death?

At first, yes. After some contemplation? Maybe. It's a lot like eating snails. Once you get comfortable with the idea, swallowing is easier.

A couple of things to consider here: (1) unless you have the hardest of hearts and/or the sparsest of resources, you are going to choose to help your parents in some way. (2) purchasing life insurance on your parents' life doesn't make them die any sooner or any later. (3) If you have expended resources that you'll need in the future to take care of your parents now, how will you rebuild them? If you have an answer that pre-empts and trumps life insurance, then use it. If not, then consider it.

As a parting note here, over the years I have seen many insurance checks delivered to widows, widowers and surviving children. While I have almost always heard them inquire whether there was any more, I have never heard them direct the agent to take some back. Think of the death proceeds not as the Great Windfall, but as the seed capital for family financial independence for generations to come. What a fantastic legacy for parents to leave: intergenerational financial independence.

REASON #20: My parents don't want to talk about their health with me but I see things that need attention.

> There are a number of reasons to talk to your parents about their health but the primary one has nothing to do with health at all.

There are a number of reasons to talk to your parents about their health but the primary one has nothing to do with health at all. It has everything to do with regulation. A new regulation, HIPPA that recently went into effect makes it virtually impossible to give, get or otherwise receive or disseminate information, about your parents' health without the appropriate documentation. You may find under HIPPA that even lifelong family physicians will be reluctant to provide information without at least something on file.

Minimally, you should get a Healthcare Power of Attorney signed. This is a sort of omnibus or master document giving broad legal powers as far as healthcare is concerned. Show up with one of these naming you as the decision authority, assuming it's properly witnessed and noticed, and you have the key to operate the healthcare conversation. Without it, you are the equivalent of the beggar at the gate.

The "I don't want to talk about healthcare" is part privacy, part protection, and all personal. Tell them that you need this to be able to get the highest care.

REASON #21: How do I know whether I can trust someone who claims to be a Parent Care Specialist to act in my best interest? Aren't they just interested in selling me some sort of financial product like long-term care insurance or life insurance?

Those are two great questions and ones you should have the answers to.

A Parent Care Specialist has been trained to go through The D.O.S. Conversation*, to gather information, and to make observations and recommendations based on individual's goals. They have been trained to charge a fee for this process so that their recommendations are:

1. Made completely at arms length
2. Able to withstand outside scrutiny as to compliancy and integrity
3. Able to allow other existing advisors to implement their recommendations.

The various regulatory agencies for life insurance, long-term care, and asset management all have very specific rules and regulations for professionals receiving compensation directly or indirectly from the sale of financial products in each one of those areas as well as disclosure forms concerning the amount of compensation received and any potential conflicts of interest.

The Parent Care Solution has been designed to remove any obligations by you to deal with any professional from any of these products. What you are purchasing from these individuals are observations and recommendations about your situation based on their years of wisdom and experience.

REASON #22: How do I know whom to trust with the management of my parents' assets once I complete *The Parent Care Solution?*

The key here is what we call the 3 C's: Character, Competence, and Capability. Let's take a look at these.

Character – fundamentally, the person and business reputation of the advisor. A quick way is to ask for a client reference, an attorney or accountant who has done business with them and someone who has first-hand knowledge of their business and personal dealings.

Competence – Basically, (1) How long have they been doing their profession (2) Who have they done work for in their profession and (3) What are their professional credentials and accomplishments that would allow you to believe they have made a career habit of professional growth and development.

Capability – Capability is really about resources both intellectually, professionally, and structurally to be able to deliver what they say they can deliver and continue to support that delivery in the foreseeable future.

Everyone that you work with should be forthright about how they are charging, what they are charging for and who is paying what fees to whom and why. More importantly, you should be receiving value in the way that you determine value no matter who is providing that service.

REASON #23: How do I know if I am receiving value in *The Parent Care Solution* for the money I am paying?

Value like beauty is often delegated functionally to the eyes of the beholder. We think there's a less ambiguous way to discern whether value is being provided. The best definition of value created we are aware of comes from The Strategic Coach Program*. Value creation comes from an individual's Unique Ability* (that thing for which they have great passion) which gives them

> Value like beauty is often delegated functionally to the eyes of the beholder.

great energy, they love doing it, and for which they have desire
to endlessly improve) Translated through:

- **Leadership** – The ability to restore confidence;
  to transform fear into focused thinking,
  communication, and action.
- **Relationship** – The ability to create, restore,
  and perpetuate confidence.
- **Creativity** – Providing flexible, acceptable,
  and evolving structures capable of meeting
  the evolving needs of people.

The by-products of leadership, relationship, and creativity are
that simplicity, balance, and the ability to focus are restored to
the situation at hand. So, the test for value is relatively simple
when you look at it from those perspectives. Are you being
provided direction in a way that helps to minimize, reduce, or
eliminate the potential for loss? Is your fear concern or
apprehension about their situation being transformed so that
you can think clearly about it, act clearly about it, and
communicate clearly about it to all those concerned? Finally, is
the structure flexible, adaptable, and innovative as it relates to
your current and future needs? If yes is the answer to about 80%
of the questions, then value seems to be there.

**REASON #24: My parents say that they can't make all these
decisions now because they weren't sure what they're going
to do and even if they were, they might change their minds?**

Well, maybe they can and then again, maybe they can't,

maybe they will and then again, maybe they won't. Neither of the two reasons above for not having the conversation really holds up under scrutiny.

The Parent Care Solution is designed through The D.O.S. Conversation* to allow your parents to determine (1) What their future looks like around long-term care whether they make the actual decisions now or later and (2) whether they trust you enough to discuss these issues with you. Until you know what their future looks like from their eyes and until you know whether they are willing to share that with you, neither you nor your parents have a real basis to go forward.

REASON #25: I have heard horror stories of children who have taken care of aging parents and who eventually regretted it because of the tremendous energy drain it required. Shouldn't I just leave this up to the professionals?

First of all resentment is a choice, not a guaranteed outcome in this situation and secondly the professional will end up taking over at some point. Unless you just completely divorce yourself emotionally from your parents, as well as physically refuse to be with them, you will be at least minimally involved with considerations about their care.

Make no mistake. Resentment over taking care of aging parents with the demands of emotional energy and financial resources can creep insidiously over time. This is exacerbated when you find yourself thrown into the middle of a parent care crisis situation.

The D.O.S. Conversation* goes a long way to diffusing the factors that lead to resentment. While admittedly an amateur in the relatively thin art of psychoanalytic theory, my sense is that people are most likely to resent situations where they are out of control, manipulated, or minimized in terms of options available and that they in turn resent the people who put them in those situations.

The D.O.S. Conversation* is the Swiss army knife of interpersonal communication tools. We have used it in numerous situations from directing care for clients to conversations about vacations with teenagers with really good conversation as the result.

> Remember that resentment usually comes because of a lack of communication, not an abundance of it.

Remember that resentment usually comes because of a lack of communication, not an abundance of it.

REASON #26: A psychologist friend of mine told me that *The Parent Care Solution* sounds like a dangerous thing in the hands of an amateur and these conversations should be conducted by trained therapists and counselors certified in these areas.

The psychological profession in the United States has invented nearly 212 syndromes, psychoses and addictions since its creation. While undoubtedly doing good work in certain situations, they would have you believe that everything involves an addiction, dependency, disorder, dysfunction or inner child of some dimension.

While the Parent Care Specialist does not have any formal psychological training nor are they trained in the various tenants of psychological theory, they are still capable of initiating and facilitating one of the most revealing and insightful psychological conversations
on the planet – The D.O.S. Conversation*.

The D.O.S. Conversation* is not about the past anything. It's all about the future. The interesting thing about the future is that in order to participate in a conversation about it with someone **(1) they have to have an idea of what it looks like for them and (2) they have to be willing to share it with you.** It doesn't require that you have extensive training in psychological process, psychiatric treatment, or family system dynamics. It just requires that you ask a series of questions and wait for the answers. The questions prompt people to think about their future. Their answers tell you what that future looks like to them along with what they are scared about, what they're excited about, and the strengths or advantages they bring to those situations.

> The D.O.S. Conversation* is not about the past anything. It's all about the future.

If professional therapists are required to have conversations with parents about parent care, my fear is that the shear numbers of conversations that will be required in the future almost guarantee there will be no conversations nor enough care.

REASON #27: I don't even know how to begin a conversation with my parents, much less continue it to find out all this stuff.

I read something once that childhood was what we spent most of our life trying to forget and it was our parents who make that impossible. So, it's only natural that going from a "What time will you be home?" conversation to a "What home will you be going to" is a bit awkward.

The D.O.S. Conversation* provides a structure to begin the conversation. Remember The D.O.S. Conversation is all about them. It's all about their future. It's about their dangers, their opportunities, and their strengths. It is human nature to want to talk about yourself and the D.O.S. Conversation allows you to do that.

Help your parents trust you with a vision of that future and then let them tell you what they are scared about, excited about, and what strengths they have to help them through it.

CHAPTER 10

The Hear and Now Listening System™

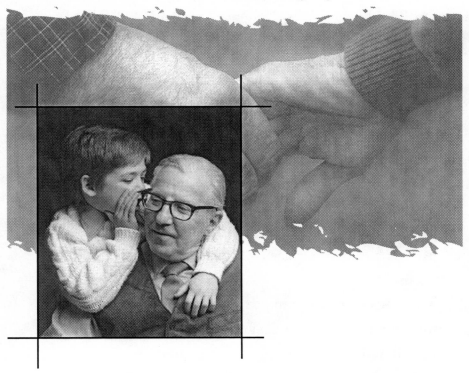

U.S. Supreme Court Justice, Potter Stewart, when once asked to define pornography, replied, "I don't know how to define it exactly, I just know it when I see it." Listening is a lot the same way. We don't know how to define it, but we know when it is present. More importantly, we are acutely aware when it isn't.

It might seem strange to have a chapter on how to listen in a book for grown-ups on how to have a conversation. The fact of the matter is that without being able to listen, the six conversations become nothing more than a set of word transactions, devoid of meaning and without content.

Nothing in the Boomer's world or their parents' has taught either of them to listen to each other or to anyone else for that matter. All around are examples of not listening as the norm. Whether it's talk TV with the hosts finishing each other's sentences, interrupting, or shouting to be heard or the cacophony of print and media competing for every centimeter of unused visual and auditory space, nothing around us gives us a way or a space to listen responsively.

> Nothing in the Boomer's world or their parents' has taught either of them to listen to each other or to anyone else for that matter.

The purpose of listening to your parents is to be able to capture the words, emotions, and reasoning of the experience they are describing as they answer the questions. What is all this experience of listening stuff? Can't you just ask the questions, get the answers and move on? You could if you were taking an online survey but here, in the six conversations you're using the questions as a way to establish connection, deepen communication and begin collaboration on a bunch of important issues.

Here's a different way to think about this listening experience process. Try to remember the last time you saw a really good film or play. You know, the type that gets you from the opening credits or beginning score and before you know it, you're part of the experience that you came to just watch. Really great films and plays create an abundance of thoughts and emotions as you move along through the storyline. Imagine how that experience would change for you if you suddenly stopped in the middle of the film and began showing a movie of your own making on top of it or sent your cast of characters on the stage with the play in progress. The experience of the original film or play is ruined and the effect is never quite achieved because of the interruption.

Listening to your parents in these conversations is a lot like the movie experience above. When people are talking they are inviting you to see and hear the movie that is going on inside their heads. By not being fully present and engaged you run the risk of missing important pieces of the story that they are trying to tell.

In the pages that follow are some thoughts and ideas about all the things that affect the way we hear and listen. The purpose of all that information is to help you create an environment where you and your parents can engage in a series of conversations that bring clarity, communication, and collaboration. It may seem awkward at first to really be present and listening. My experience has shown that parents really want to be listened to more than you can imagine. Especially concerning the topics that these conversations ask them to consider.

Listening in *The Parent Care Conversation* is a three dimensional, physical, emotional, intellectual experience. It is both watching a movie and listening to a book on tape. It requires asking questions to solve a mystery and responding in a way that encourages communication but at the same time stays the course. It is being present at such a level of intensity that one actually feels as if they were being complimented.

My Buddhist friends say that the greatest gift one can give is that of attention. Attention has as its implication the process of being present; of being here in the moment, centered, focused, as calm as one can be while using words, gestures and other actions that communicate as closely as possible how it is you feel and what it is that you want. What you want, ultimately want, as the listener, is for the storyteller to fully and completely convey all that is desired to be conveyed; not only to be heard but to be understood, to verify as well as value, to gather and to glean. Sounds like some tough requirements just to have a conversation. Well, if they do it's because they are.

There is great power in listening and being listened to. Psychologically when we listen our heart rate and oxygen consumption are reduced. Our blood pressure is decreased and we have the feeling of being empowered by new energy. Intellectually and emotionally, listening is the very first step in creating value for someone. In The Strategic Coach Program* , value is defined as our Unique Ability* to bring leadership, relationship and creativity to a situation. Leadership is always about direction for someone. That leadership can be eliminating dangers from the situation or

> Leadership is always about direction for someone.

pointing the way to opportunities that people may overlook or be unable to see how they can take advantage of.

Relationship is always about confidence. In the series entitled, "Always Increase Your Confidence*", confidence is the ability to transform fear into focused and directed thinking, communication and action in such a way as weaknesses become strengths, obstacles become innovations, and setbacks become breakthroughs. The confidence element is absolutely essential in paving the way to a successful conversation because one cannot take in new information if confidence is low. Nor can we act on information if confidence is low. *The Parent Care Solution* is designed to constantly increase the confidence of the participants by helping them to focus on the future, which increases energy, gaining control of all of the details of their affairs, which restores simplicity and reduces complexity and making their decisions in a holistic, integrated manner which restores balance. The end result is that their focus is restored in designing a solution instead of analyzing the past or agonizing about the future.

Creativity comes in the form of designing structures and options that are capable of being adaptable and flexible as situations change or evolve. *The Parent Care Solution* is a highly creative structure designed to maintain complete control over the design and outcome of one's decisions in a very complicated and complex time for the majority of people.

Experts in the field of listening suggest that there is both active and passive listening, that there are states that are more involved than others. Our experience has shown that in some ways these distinctions are meaningless. It is like saying that you are either actively watching a movie or passively watching a movie. That is ridiculous. Either you are watching a movie or you are not. You are engaged or you are not. Listening is exactly the same thing.

When people are talking they are asking you in a way to become a part of their movie. The difficulty comes when you choose to not watch their's by disconnecting in some way or, worse yet, by attempting to project your movie over theirs.

In *The Parent Care Solution*, there is only listening or not listening. You are either present or you are not. If you are listening, the speaker will in most cases tell you exactly what you need to go on to the next decision. If you are not listening, you will miss the information that you need to make that next step. In order to know whether you are listening or not, or better yet, whether it is possible to listen or not depending on distractions from inside your listening equipment (head) or outside (the room) the equipment needs to be tuned in and facilitating the listening.

> The potential for miscommunication and misinformation is staggering…

In terms of the structures that affect listening, there are any number that singularly and acting in concert, either encourage or discourage really beneficial listening. The physical room; the type, manner and order of questions; the rhythm and pacing of the conversation structure;

the semantics, tone and intent of the words; the syntactic structure; and the structure of repetition, all encourage or discourage, facilitate or inhibit listening.

The potential for miscommunication and misinformation is staggering when we consider that of the 800,000 estimated words in the English language, we use only 800 of them fairly consistently. Of those 800, we have at least 15-17 meanings per word. Conservatively, if everything else is working, we have a 1 in 17 chance of being misunderstood. This is further complicated when we realize that 55% of what we communicate is communicated non-verbally with gestures, facial expressions, eyebrows and eyes, 38% by voice tone, rhythm and pacing. Only 7% of what we actually communicate is accomplished by words.

So, what is the remaining 93% about? It is about being present, being attentive and being aware to the answers in all of the Parent Care Conversations.

Just as the music is found between the notes in great symphonies, the meaning in our parents' life is a symphony of sight and sound and experience. Make sure you listen to their great music.

Your Parent Care Solution

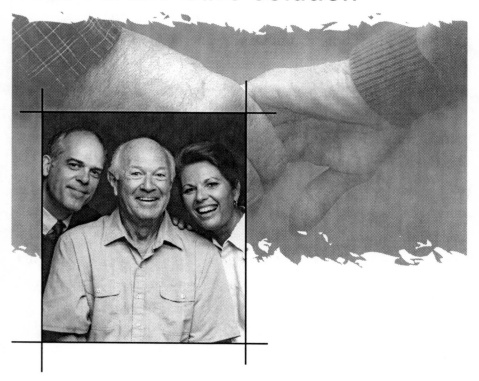

So you might ask, after reading all of this, what are all these conversations for and who really cares if I have them or not? Why not just go along and let things sort themselves out as they happen? All this talk and information is really a lot of work and doesn't avoid what's going to happen anyway: parents are going to get older, get sicker, and spend their final days in a strange place, cared for by strange people urinating in flower vases and looking for their car keys...or will they?

I can't tell you that having the Parent Care Conversations prevents any of those things. At the time of this writing my father is entering his fourth year in the Special Care Ward of Brighton Gardens becoming unable to button his shirt, wash his own hair, or remember whether he's had lunch or not. During the times I visit with him I watch his struggle to line up the words to make thoughts inside his head so that sentences come out. I am aware of the toll this struggle has taken on me, I can only imagine the price it has exacted from him.

The Parent Care Solution really does nothing to prevent any of those things happening to him or anyone else who uses it. *The Parent Care Solution* doesn't prevent cancer, arthritis, Lou Gehrig's, or Parkinson's disease. It can't create wealth where there is none nor can it prevent the spending of it all if that's what the care requires. It cannot make 100% happy what is at times 1,000 percent sad. It cannot do anything to prevent some of the inevitabilities of simply getting older.

But here's what it can do for you. It can begin a series of conversations that over time increase the quality of a great parent-child relationship and perhaps begin one that needs to begin.

It allows us to decide things together with our parents that we cannot begin to contemplate apart. It allows us to paint a picture of their life past, present, and future that creates a context in which we all can be connected. In short, it just may help us to make sense of it all.

What *The Parent Care Solution* really provides to you is a relationship tool that begins with the mechanics of money and ends with conversations about the meaning. Along the way something happens to everyone involved. I believe what happens is that we gain clarity, and connection with the people that provided the canvas that provided the background on which the portraits of our own lives were painted.

The Parent Care Solution allows us to say the things we've always wanted to say now, instead of waiting for the memorial service. The paradox in obituaries and eulogies is not that they are meaningless because they aren't. The paradox is that the one who could've benefited the most from them isn't available to listen.

The Parent Care Solution provides the opportunity for a spiritual connection that many parent-child relationships would like to experience but don't know how. On any given day my sense of the eternal ranges from Woody Allen's belief that "all souls go to a garage near Buffalo" to Emerson's more existential view that "we sit in the lap of an immense intelligence". My own definition is even narrower; it is simply the way we relate to each other as human beings; how we talk with each other, support each other, encourage each other and protect each other. It is all about helping each other constantly and consistently see and shape our future, overcome our fears, maximize our opportunities and take advantage of all the advantages we have.

The Parent Care Solution allows you to move from being a

member of the audience in your family theater to a participant on the stage. This transition creates a change in perspective that is truly unique.

As I participate and watch in what appears to be the final act in an incredible play called "My Father's Life", I am struck with how the design of that play makes the roles transferable for me and those who would come after. Shakespeare's insight that "all the world's a stage with each of us required to play a part" seems particularly prophetic these days.

As I have made the journey from money to meaning with my father, I have become aware of how quickly we go from having no time for conversation to having all the time but no conversation. I am more thankful than ever for all the great conversations my father and I had.

My wish for you is that *The Parent Care Solution* provides an opportunity for the greatest of conversations with those whom you should have the greatest of conversations… Don't you dare miss the conversations.

The Parent Care Solution Tools

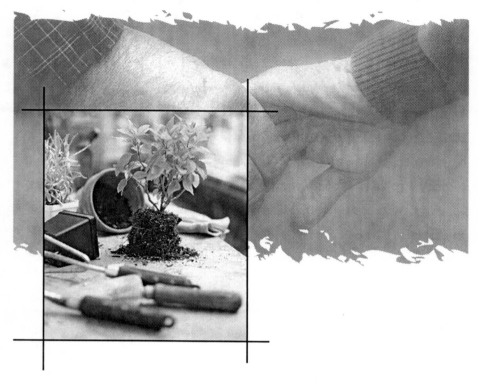

The Parent Care Solution Tools™ are my devices for helping you make decisions in some pretty important areas. Whether it is evaluating an advisor, getting a house ready for sale, or deciding which source of money to use first, I hope these are as quick and easy as I intended. I hope they will be as helpful to you as they have been for me.

THE ADVISOR ESSENTIAL QUESTIONS™

1. What is your primary business?

2. How long have you been doing it?

3. What have you achieved professionally?

4. Who do I know who knows you?

5. What would your most favorite client say about you?

6. What would your least favorite client say about you?

7. Would it be possible to talk with either of them?

8. Tell me how you would see us working together?

9. How do you see that you would become better by working with me?

10. How will my situation improve if we work together?

11. Is there anything you should tell me about yourself that if I found out later, it would be disappointing?

12. Will I be working with you, an associate, or your team?

13. What do you estimate will be your annual compensation from working with me?

14. How accessible and available are you realistically?

15. Is there anything you would like to ask me?

SOURCES

National Association of Personal Financial Advisors www.napfa.org

Certified Financial Planner Board of Standards www.cfp.net

THE DOCUMENT DIRECTORY CHECKLIST™

FOR: _____

The following information should be easily located and accessible to the holder of your power of attorney. Complete account numbers, phone numbers and addresses should be noted whenever possible.

DOCUMENT	DONE	DATE	LOCATION
CPA			
Lawyer			
Auto Title			
Home Title			
Deeds			
Bank Account			
Brokerage Accounts			
Credit Card Accounts			
Employer Information			
Insurance Agent			
Insurance Policies			
Medicare, Medicaid or Health Insurance Cards			
Pastor, Minister, Priest, or Rabbi			
Mortgage Papers			
Passport			
Physicians			
Dentists			
Opthamologist			
Social Security			
Investment Advisor			
Financial Planner			
Banker			
General Power of Attorney			
Healthcare Power of Attorney			

THE IMPORTANT DOCUMENTS TIME LINE™

DOCUMENT	HOW LONG?	WHY?
Tax Return	6 Years	IRS can audit within 3 years if they suspect a filing error. Same applies if you file an amended return. IRS has six years for 25% understatement of income.
Cancelled Checks	6 Years	Just because.
Brokerage Statements Mutual Funds Bank Statements	6 Years	Same as IRS; for IRS back-up.
Real Estate	6 Years	IRS back-up.
Paycheck Stubs	6 Years	IRS back-up. Also save final pay stub of year for cumulative withholding information.
Credit Card Statements	6 Years	IRS back-up especially if business purchases have been made.
Retirement Plan Data	6 Years	Quarterly statments until end of year; the annual statement.

THE HOUSE REPAIR CHECKLIST™

Most contracts for sale require that an inspection be made and accepted by the buyer prior to sale. To avoid surprises, consider checking into the following before putting your parents' home on the market.

ITEM	FAIR	GOOD	EXCELLENT	REPAIR	ESTIMATE
Roof Quality					
Windows					
Frames					
Sills					
Doors					
Frames					
Locks					
Body					
Walls					
Paint					
Plaster					
Wall Coverings					
HVAC					
Plumbing					
Kitchen					
Bath					
Bath					
Exterior					
Fencing					
Guttering					
Sprinkler System					
Appliances					
Refrigerator					
Stove					
Microwave					
Insulation					
Pavement					
Tiling					
Patio					
Pool					
Electrical					
Indoor					
Outdoor					

HOUSE REPAIR RESOURCES

American Institute of Architects
> 800-242-3837
> www.aiaccess.com

Contractors
> Check with State Boards for all
> projects over $500. They are
> required to have a license.

Handymen
> The Handyman Connection
> www.handymanconnection.com

Interior Designers
> American Society of Interior
> Designers (ASID)
> 800-755-2743
> www.interiors.org

Remodelers
> Division of National Association
> of Homebuilders
> 800-223-2665
> www.nahb.org

Repairmen
> Service Magic
> www.servicemagic.com
> Check out their "Project Estimator"
> help ad.

THE PROPERTY DECISION SYSTEM™

Current Location				
Piece of Property				
Description				
Approximate Value				
Prior Decisions	Yes	To Whom?	Do They Know?	How?
	Date			
Prior Decisions	No	To Whom?	By What Way?	
	When?			

What does this mean to me?

What do I want it to mean to the person who receives it?

Who else might enjoy this if my first choice is unwilling or incapable of accepting it?

How do I want this resolved if there is a dispute?

What is my ultimate dispute resolving wish?

THE PROPERTY DECISION SYSTEM™

FIRST FLOOR	WHERE STORED?	WHEN?	BY WHOM?
Foyer			
Hallway			
Living Room			
Den			
Kitchen			
Great Room			
Closet			
Bath			
Laundry Room			

THE PROPERTY DECISION SYSTEM™

SECOND FLOOR	WHERE STORED?	WHEN?	BY WHOM?
Foyer			
Hallway			
Bedroom #1			
Bedroom #2			
Bedroom #3			
Bedroom #4			
Bedroom #5			
Bedroom #6			
Bath #1			
Bath #2			
Bath #3			
Linen Closet			

THE PROPERTY DECISION SYSTEM™

THIRD FLOOR	WHERE STORED?	WHEN?	BY WHOM?
Hallway			
Bedroom #1			
Bedroom #2			
Bath			
Linen Closet			

GARAGE	WHERE STORED?	WHEN?	BY WHOM?

BASEMENT	WHERE STORED?	WHEN?	BY WHOM?

ATTIC	WHERE STORED?	WHEN?	BY WHOM?

OTHER	WHERE STORED?	WHEN?	BY WHOM?

THE PROPERTY DECISION SYSTEM™

PERSONAL ITEMS	WHERE STORED?	WHEN?	BY WHOM?
Jewelry			
Art			
Antiques			
Watches			
Tangibles			

THE EXPENSE SYSTEM™

INCOME		Charitable	
Salary		Hobbies	
Bonus		Child Care	
Freelance		Pets	
Social Security		Auto Loan	
Pension		Auto Expense	
Annuity Income		Oil	
Interest		Gas	
Dividends		Repair	
Other		Auto Registration	
		Public Transportation	
EXPENSES		Interest	
Home		Non-Reimbursable/Med. Bills	
Mortgage/Rent		Legal Fees	
HE Loan		Accounting Fees	
Property Taxes		Credit Card Payments	
Condo/Co-op Fees			
Home Owner Dues		INSURANCE	
Utilities		Health	
Phone		Dental	
Gas		Life	
Electric		Disability	
Fuel		Doctor Visits	
Water		Medicare	
Cable		Eyeglasses	
Repairs/Home Expense		Prescriptions	
Upkeep			
Furniture		TAXES	
Day to Day		Federal	
Food		State	
Liquor		Local	
Dining Out		Self-Employment	
Clothing		Other	
Cosmetics			
Entertainment		TOTAL EXPENSES	
Gym		TOTAL INCOME	
Gifts		SURPLUS/DEFICIT	

THE EASY MONEY/HARD MONEY DECISIONS™

EASY MONEY		HARD MONEY	
Cash on Hand		Real Estate Equity	
Checking Accounts		Tangibles	
Certificates of Deposit		Art	
Money Market Accounts		Antiques	
Stock Mutual Funds		Jewelry	
Bond Mutual Funds		Rare coins	
Individual Stocks		Collectibles	
Individual Bonds		Heirlooms	
Annuities		Pension Plan	
Cash-Value Life Insurance		Profit Sharing Plans	
Gifts		SEP	
		SIMPLE	
		401-K	
		Other Qualified Plan	
		Loans	
		Reverse Mortgage	
		Line of Credit	
TOTAL EASY MONEY		TOTAL HARD MONEY	

Steps for Easy Money Analysis

1. Total all the Easy Money amounts.

2. Divide the total by the monthly amount required.

3. Determine number of months available.

Steps for Hard Money Analysis

1. Total all the Hard Money amounts.

2. Divide the total by the monthly amount required.

3. Determine number of months available.

Total # of Easy Money months plus total # Hard Money months equals total number of care months available.

THE CARE FACILITY CRITICAL QUESTIONS™

1. What impression do the buildings and grounds create?
2. Is the floorplan easy to understand and follow?
3. Are all important rooms of the facility wheelchair accessible?
4. Are elevators and ramps for the physically challenged available?
5. Are all essential shelves, closets and storage easy to reach?
6. Are all surfaces non-skid and all floor coverings securely fastened?
7. Is there an abundance and a balance of natural and artificial lighting?
8. Is the facility clean and fresh smelling as well as free of odors?
9. Are heating and air conditioning units capable of handling individual and facility demands?
10. Are hand rails installed in appropriate places such as hallways and individual bath units?
11. Are there clear fire and emergency escape plans with clearly marked exits?
12. Is the facility financially solvent?
13. Is the facility adequately staffed and are all staff licensed in good standing with regulatory agencies?
14. Is there a registered dietician or other nutrition expert on staff?
15. Does the facility maintain in-house 24-hour nurse on call availability or physician on call? What is the response time?
16. Who or what provides emergency physician services?
17. How close is the facility to the nearest acute care hospital or trauma center? What is the response time?
18. Does the facility offer a written plan of care capable of flexibility and adaptability for the residents changing needs?
19. Do the programs qualify for government, corporate, or private programs to help cover service cost?
20. Do the residents appear to have some degree of privacy and access to quiet and calm surroundings?
21. Are all required licenses current and on display?
22. Is a Patients Bill of Rights posted in plain sight?
23. Are there daily or weekly social functions or activities available to the residents?
24. Is the facility under investigation by any agency or has it been cited for violations in the past?
25. Is this where you want your parent to be and do you want to visit them here?

RESOURCES TO LOCATE A FACILITY

Retirement Living Information Center
> 203-938-0417
> www.retirementliving.com

Senior Resource
> 877-793-7901
> www.seniorresource.com

American Association of Homes and Services for the Aging
> 202-783-2242
> www.aahsa.org
> 202-783-2243

Adult 55+ Communities
> 877-55-ACTIVE
> www.activeadulthousing.com

Covenant Retirement Communities
> 800-255-8989
> www.covenantretirement.com

Webb Active Adult Communities
> 800-808-8088
> www.delwebb.com

ACKNOWLEDGEMENTS

It would have been impossible to write this book without the contributions along the way from the following people. I am indebted to them way into the future for their work.

Brian Carroll, Glenn Main, and **Mark Patterson** for spending a day in a Pittsburgh hotel room waiting patiently as I outlined *The Parent Care Solution* concept and for their continuing collaboration. Specifically:

Mark Patterson for his graphic interpretation of *The Parent Care Solution* concept and his ongoing branding support.

Glenn Main for his wisdom and insight into the insurance industry and its current state of affairs. Also, thanks to Glenn for being my classmate and partner in Coach2.

Brian Carroll, my partner, attorney, caregiver and advisor extraordinaire.

C. Timothy Hodge, my partner and friend for his consistent marketing of *The Parent Care Solution* into organizations and institutions that wouldn't have recorded that I called, much less returned them.

Donald Taylor, my brother and promoter extraordinaire of the entire concept. He believes in me even when he doesn't like me.

The Strategic Coach Inc., **Dan Sullivan** and his partner, **Babs Smith** for without their incredible program, Coach2 and their increasing wisdom and experience, none of this would have been possible. Special thanks to **Ross Slater** and **Catherine Nomura,** The Strategic Coach Intellectual Capital team who made licensing and creation a terrific experience. All companies in the world would do well by observing how this company deals with the world and more importantly how it is transforming it.

Vince Quattrini, attorney and Strategic Coach* client who besides being one of the premier social security and workers compensation attorneys in the country, gave me extremely valuable insights and feedback from beginning to end. I am proud to be his business friend and even more fortunate to share in his wisdom.

Scott Fischer at Fischer Capital. What do you say about someone whose presence made your opportunity a reality? My admiration, respect and gratitude for the rest of my time.

Mark Bass of Pennington Bass, Lubbock, Texas. Besides being one of the top financial advisors in the country, he has been invaluable in reviewing the various drafts and options as we created the book. He is my best friend and my hope is to be half the advisor and human being that he is.

The Special Care Staff at Brighton Gardens, Charlotte, North Carolina.

Christine Sheffield, my life partner of 11 years who has typed manuscripts, created brochures, answered telephones and generally made all the creative part of my life possible while at the same time raising her daughter, Ashley, and helping me take care of my father. My thanks forever.

The dogs: **Katy, Roxanne** and **Zack** who are always by my side, always glad to see me, always ready with a sloppy kiss and more than willing to plunge into the pool on writing breaks. I only hope heaven has a place for creatures like this. It will be a better eternity if they're there.

Finally, **my dad** – What do you say about someone who made all of my life possible? He made my life an exceptional multiple of what his was... he always fought the good fight, always kept the faith and always finished the race no matter how arduous. The world and I are better because he was in it.

The poet **Emily Dickinson** may not have been thinking of Alzheimer's when she penned the following lines, but I think they apply nicely to those of us contemplating our aging parents:

> *"My life closed twice before its close*
> *and it yet remains to see*
> *If immortality shall reveal*
> *A third event to me.*
> *So huge, so hopeless to conceive.*
> *All these that twice befell.*
> *Parting is all we know of heaven*
> *And all we need of hell."*

You may order copies of
The Parent Care Solution
in paperback or e-book
directly from our website:
www.parentcaresolution.com

Printed in the United States
105269LV00004B/5/A